More Acclaim for *Ticker*

"A fast-paced, utterly riveting tale of the decades of effort that have gone i̇
developing an artificial heart. The characters, many of whom dedicated the
lives to this quest, are captivating, and their rivalries are the stuff of legend."
—Bethany McLean, coauthor of *All the Devils Are Here* and
The Smartest Guys in the Room

"A remarkable journey through the harrowing world of heart surgery, as a bril-
liantly gifted and eccentric team of doctors work to develop a complete artificial
heart to save the thousands of patients a year whose hearts are failing."
—Bryan Burrough, author of *Public Enemies*, *The Big Rich*, and
Barbarians at the Gate

"An exciting, propulsive, and at times surprisingly tender account of the swash-
buckling surgeons and inventive geniuses who are working to achieve one of the
greatest medical breakthroughs—the development of the artificial heart. Mimi
Swartz has done an outstanding job and uncovered the human story behind the
triumph of technology."
—Jennet Conant, *New York Times* bestselling author of *Tuxedo Park* and
109 East Palace

"Who knew that the story of the artificial heart was such a rip-roaring one, with
one larger-than-life character after another, and plot twists galore? In *Ticker*,
Mimi Swartz has told that story with verve and elegance, and brought those
characters to vivid life. A wonderful work of nonfiction by a wonderful nonfiction writer."
—Joe Nocera, *Bloomberg News* columnist and author of *Indentured:*
The Inside Story of the Rebellion Against the NCAA

TICKER

TICKER

THE QUEST TO CREATE AN ARTIFICIAL HEART

MIMI SWARTZ

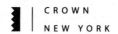

CROWN
NEW YORK

Library of Congress Cataloging-in-Publication Data
Names: Swartz, Mimi, author.
Title: Ticker : the quest to create an artificial heart / Mimi Swartz.
Description: New York : Crown, [2018] | Includes bibliographical
    references and index.
Identifiers: LCCN 2017058910 | ISBN 9780804138000
    (hardback) | ISBN 9780804138017 (ebook)
Subjects: | MESH: Frazier, O. Howard. | Cohn, Billy. | Heart,
    Artificial | Surgeons | United States
Classification: LCC RD598.35.T7 | NLM WG 169.5 |
    DDC 617.4/120592—dc23 LC record available at
    https://lccn.loc.gov/2017058910

ISBN 978-0-8041-3800-0
Ebook ISBN 978-0-8041-3801-7

Printed in the United States of America

Jacket design by Christopher Brand
Jacket photograph: The Voorhes

10 9 8 7 6 5 4 3 2 1

First Edition

To my father, husband, and son
Who taught me the most important lessons of the human heart

Diseases desperate grown
By desperate appliance are relieved,
Or not at all.

—WILLIAM SHAKESPEARE, *Hamlet,* Act 4, Scene 3

"How about my heart?" asked the Tin Woodman.

"Why, as for that," answered Oz, "I think you are wrong to want a heart. It makes most people unhappy. If you only knew it, you are in luck not to have a heart."

"That must be a matter of opinion," said the Tin Woodman. "For my part, I will bear all the unhappiness without a murmur, if you will give me the heart."

—FRANK BAUM, *The Wizard of Oz*

CONTENTS

TICKER

THE TIN MAN

The kids fell in love with him first. Craig Lewis lived three houses down, a tall, solitary beanpole of a man with a copper-colored golden retriever named Shogun. He looked to be in his late thirties, and Linda Sanders knew from neighborhood gossip that he had one marriage behind him, just like she did. Back then, Shogun seemed to be his constant companion. Craig had taught that dog to do just about anything—of course he could sit, stay, fetch, and hunt, but he also knew how to play hide-and-seek with even the canniest kid. That was why, as soon as Linda Sanders' children heard Craig's pickup pull into his driveway in the early evenings, they were out the door—Leslie was eight and Eddie six, two towheads on the run, raising small clouds of dust as their feet slapped the parched summer grass. "Don't wear out your welcome!" Linda warned to the screen door they slammed behind them. The sky would turn dusky and the shadows grow long before she'd give up waiting for their return and head down after them.

The last light of day was at her back, heating her neck and shoulders, and the hot, damp closeness of a Houston summer took her in its seasonal embrace. There were people who swore it always cooled off at night here, but Linda knew better. She'd lived all her life in this tattered north Houston neighborhood, and she knew what changed and what didn't, or couldn't.

Linda could see from the flattened grass that her kids had literally beaten a path to Craig's door. It was natural that they'd go looking for a man to replace the one who'd left them. Craig was handy, that was for sure: when Eddie dragged his broken bike to his door, he fixed the chain, cleaning it up with WD40. He let Leslie draw in his old sketchbooks. If the kids were talking about the moon or stars, he would haul out his telescope and let them look through it at the night sky. Once, when Linda's air conditioner broke down—the worst thing that could happen in the middle of a Houston summer—Craig came over and fixed it for her, no charge.

A slight woman of twenty-seven, Linda had a smile that was both knowing and tentative. Her thin brown hair fell lank below her shoulders. Like this street—small frame houses guarded by rusting cyclone fences—she could have been pretty if she fixed herself up, but who had the money or the time? She had been divorced for several years and was barely making ends meet as a clerk at an auto parts store. She lived with the kids in a tired two-bedroom house she rented from her mom, its sunny yellow hue fading to a peaked sunrise. Home improvements were out of the question: Leslie and Eddie were always needing new shoes, school clothes, tetanus shots, whatever. Every day seemed like the one before it: get up, get the kids out the door to school, get them home, do homework, feed them dinner, then give them baths, put them to bed, and get up and do it all over again. She was in her late twenties, going on forty-five.

Maybe that's why she found Craig's place such a comfort. Her front yard could have been mistaken for a small daycare center, with the kids' toys and bikes scattered all over the place; his was manicured and trimmed. Wanting to get out of the sun, she pushed his door open, something Craig had told her she was welcome to do.

Neat as a pin inside and out, she thought. Craig was a project manager for the city—he had walked away from community college just shy of graduation because he didn't see the point, he had told her. The engineers with the big degrees started calling him for advice after his first few months on the job anyway. He was teaching Leslie to fold clothes—he towered over the little girl as they did that funny laundry waltz in the living room with the sheet getting smaller and smaller between them. Leslie was giggling, the corners of the bedsheet clutched between her stubby fingers. Linda looked around for Eddie, scanning the glossy wooden floor, the sofa still peppy and full from disuse, the walls lined with bookcases filled with volumes on engineering and medicine and oil field equipment. No sign of him.

She looked at Craig quizzically, and he met her gaze, and for just a moment she caught a twinkle in his eyes. Then he turned away. "Shogun, find Eddie," he said to the dog, who had been sitting, attentive, as if waiting for the command. In a flash Shogun dashed into the kitchen, where he skidded to the front of a cabinet door. Then, with a sigh, he dropped to the ground, beating his tail on the hard floor, moving his eyes from the handle to Craig and back again, waiting. Craig bent over to take the final fold of the sheet from Leslie, and put a finger to his lips. Then he stepped toward the dog and threw the cabinet doors open to reveal Eddie, crouched over like a beach ball.

"I'll spoil your dog if you'll train my kids," Linda told him. She shooed them toward the front door, patting them between their shoulder blades both to hurry them along and to claim them as hers.

That was how Craig and Linda started spending time together. She'd rent a video and then pass it on to him, since they were good for two days. If she made extra for dinner, she'd take him a plate. Once, the kids locked her out of the house and she had to go to him for help to get back in. Craig came down, took the sliding door out, put it back in, and then gave her a stick to put at the base to keep robbers away. He was around so much, in fact, that Linda's mom started including him when she dropped by with ice-cream sandwiches.

Taking the kids home, she thought that nothing makes a man more handsome than acting in a fatherly way with kids. Linda decided to do a little investigating. She found out that he was dating someone. Well, he'd never said anything to her about it, but that was that.

—⌇—

Then Linda met a man and moved with him and the kids to Seattle for nearly a year before she realized her mistake. When she moved back to her mom's house, Craig had disappeared. She tried to find him—babbling to the new tenant in his house about Shogun—but didn't have any luck. One night, she was playing pool and who should walk into the bar but Craig himself. They made a date to catch up. He invited the whole family to his new house and rented a video of the original *101 Dalmatians*. The kids had never seen it, he remembered. He also remembered that they loved his chicken-and-egg fajitas, which he loaded onto their plates before they all sat down on the couch to watch. "Craig, can you marry my mom?" Leslie asked. Well, Linda thought, if he had any interest, two pushy kids could put an end to things before they started.

That was okay, she told herself. After Seattle she had put her heart on the shelf, deciding to raise her kids alone. But then Craig bought the kids roller skates, and they all went skating in the park. He took them fishing. But the thing Craig loved most was to go out to dinner and then hit the Brown Book Shop, his favorite place in the world. It was where all the engineers and doctors and lawyers bought their technical books for school, a homely spot just north of the medical center, with fluorescent lights and stacks and stacks of books, a place he could lose and find himself at the same time. "Baby, these books don't have any pictures," she'd tease. She thought Craig was the smartest man she'd ever met.

They got married at the courthouse on October 15, 1993. She was thirty, he was thirty-six. "Should we bring the kids?" she asked the night before. "Of course," he said. "I'm marrying them too." Their wedding gift to each other was a hand-cranked ice-cream maker.

She felt as though she had married a man who could do anything. When he spied her recipe cards scattered in a kitchen drawer, he made Linda a recipe box out of soft yellow pine. He and Eddie built a boat together. Craig couldn't do anything halfway: first the garage and then the house began to fill up with his projects. When he got interested in chemical reactions, he bought himself a used centrifuge. He'd been a welder back in the day; now he bought himself an anvil and a forge.

Easter came. It was the prettiest time of year in Houston, when the air was still cool, the skies were a clear baby blue, and the azaleas bloomed in a riot of pink and purple and white. Before she married Craig, Linda had always planned egg hunts for her kids, buying them fancy baskets and hiding clues in plastic eggs that led them to the treasure—more plastic Easter eggs filled with quarters. That was not enough for Craig. He sent her out to buy something called a landscaping compass. The night before Easter, once the kids were asleep, he took a flashlight and spray-painted a grid in the yard. The next morning, he had the kids find their eggs by looking through the compass and following coordinates.

That was how it was for seventeen years.

"I think there might be something wrong with my heart," Craig told her one morning while he was getting dressed for work. He said it the way he said everything—calmly, like she shouldn't worry. It was September 2010; Craig was fifty-three and had never had a sick day in his life. His dad had lived to ninety-one, and his mother was still fit at eighty-nine. He could outrace the kids on bike rides no matter how fast they pedaled. But now he couldn't sleep, he was waking up nights to the pounding of his heart, like it was going to jump out of his chest. Craig made an appointment with a cardiologist, who didn't find a thing.

So Craig went back to doing what he'd always done, which at that time meant going to work during the week and keeping himself busy on weekends installing hardwood floors in their living room. But instead of staying up reading late into the night, he'd fall into bed early, exhausted.

"I'm tired," he told her.

"Well," she said, "you should be tired. I'm forty-seven and I'm tired." But really, she wasn't tired, and she didn't think he should be either.

—\/\/\—

By October, the heat was beginning to recede, giving way to that sweet, gentle coolness that can make even the most jaded Houstonian feel grateful. But Craig's racing heart continued to keep him up at night; he reminded Linda of a zombie sometimes when he got himself ready for work. Then the rash appeared. It started near an ankle, winding up his body like a snake: angry scabs of dark red that seemed to erupt from something deep under the skin.

On Thanksgiving Day 2010, Linda got up before dawn to put in the turkey, and heard Craig wheezing in bed. He had caught the cold Leslie had brought home from school, and hadn't been able to sleep at all for the last few days. Linda walked back into their bedroom, took one look at her husband's ashen face, and stripped off her nightgown and threw on a T-shirt and jeans. "We're going to the emergency room," she declared.

The highway was nearly empty owing to the holiday, and Linda flew past the billboards, pine trees, and downtown towers without a glance, craning her neck for a first glimpse of the Texas Medical Center. "You all right, baby?" she asked, but Craig wasn't up to talking. The fifteen-mile trip to St. Luke's Hospital was a blur.

In the emergency room, a doctor put a stethoscope to Craig's chest and didn't seem too worried. Probably bronchitis. They should see a pulmonologist just to rule out the beginnings of asbestosis or emphysema. Craig and Linda left with a referral and a round of antibiotics. Craig ate his turkey late that night, in bed.

Over the next few days he rallied. The color came back into his cheeks, and he got out of bed to attend to some of his projects. But then the antibiotics stopped working, and his symptoms came back worse than before. Linda called the doctor at St. Luke's again, but this time he was not quite as reassuring. "I think something more is going on," he said carefully. He prescribed another round of antibiotics—stronger ones—and urged Linda to get Craig to a pulmonologist as soon as possible. Certainly right after the holidays.

Then, just after Christmas, Craig asked her to take a look at his ankles. Looking down at the swollen flesh, Linda was reminded of the book of Job, which she'd studied in Sunday school. The swelling in his legs was getting worse every day, and by New Year's Craig couldn't walk. This time he went to St. Luke's by ambulance, and late that night he went into respiratory failure.

St. Luke's was a private hospital—Craig had good insurance through his job with the city—so the waiting room in the ER where Linda sat was almost empty when a doctor came to find her. He was wearing scrubs, and Linda could tell by the stony look on his face and the speed of his stride that he was angry.

He started yelling at her from six feet away. "How can you say your husband doesn't have heart problems?" he demanded.

"He doesn't," she said. But her voice wasn't as firm as she would have liked. She was confused.

Craig had septic shock and double pneumonia, and worse, his heart was barely beating. How could she not have known? Why had she waited so long to get him to the hospital? Seeing the confusion on her face, the doctor took a long, slow breath and softened his voice.

"Maybe he didn't tell you?" he asked.

Linda listened, trying as hard as she could to pay attention even though her mind was racing. Craig was very, very sick, he began. He had only a fifty-fifty chance of making it through the night. The doctor promised to do whatever he could to keep him alive, but he wasn't sure that he could.

The nurses let her into the cardiac ICU for just a few minutes that night, long enough for her to put a hand to Craig's forehead and push some strands of hair away. Then Linda bent toward him and whispered in her husband's ear: "You'd better wake up and tell me what I need to know."

—⋀⋀—

Dr. Oscar Howard Frazier—known to all as Bud—was a tall, broad, vigorous man who had spent so many nights on the exhausted leather sofa in his office at Houston's Texas Heart Institute that he no longer noticed it couldn't even provide a semblance of comfort. Nor did he note that his once beautiful Oriental rug, having suffered from decades of neglect, had curdled over the years to a shade somewhere between dingy beige and dingy gray. He *had* noticed that he had severely depleted the emergency wardrobe he kept in a small closet in his windowless, book-lined office—a small collection of expensive ties and elegant jackets that mostly stayed in dry cleaner bags—but he didn't have time to run home for more. Anyway, he didn't need them on this day: he had his blue-green St. Luke's hospital scrubs, which he wore over an orange and white University of Texas T-shirt. The head of the longhorn, UT's beloved mascot, peeked out from beneath the neckline.

Bud's piercing eyes were never quite visible behind the glare of his round, horn-rimmed glasses. At seventy, he had a leonine mane of shimmering white hair and the unlined, luminous skin that came from spending the better part of fifty years indoors at the hospital. The same was true of his hands: they were as large as a farm boy's and as free of age spots. Bud had also maintained an authentic West Texas drawl; he sounded to some like LBJ on Quaaludes. He lumbered a little, sometimes with a hitch in his step, the price of a high school football career in West Texas, along with years of standing for hours in the operating room. He had had four back operations, needed knee surgery but kept putting it off. Most people on the street might have taken him for a college history professor emeritus instead of a world-famous cardiac surgeon, one who had done more heart transplants than anyone else on earth—thirteen hundred, to be specific. Bud, like so many surgeons, kept count.

By the time Craig Lewis wound up in Bud's care, the patient looked like he had been incarcerated for a very long time in a prisoner of war camp. Craig had never taken the doctor's advice to see a specialist. His hospital visit following Christmas of 2010 lasted twenty-one days. He was diagnosed with multiple organ failure. One of Bud's colleagues tried to save him by putting a device called a balloon pump in his aorta to help his circulation; a kidney specialist put him on dialysis. The following Friday, Craig coded—his heart stopped, and it took a team of frantic hospital personnel to get it started again.

Bud was called in at the recommendation of another surgeon. He examined Craig and found him a challenge: the walls of his heart were too damaged for a traditional heart pump, something called a left ventricular assist device that was often used in such cases. LVADs, as they were called, were Bud's specialty and over the decades had become a popular option for the very sick; one small machine could take over the entire function of the left side of the heart, the side that did the heavy lifting, keeping the blood circulating throughout the body. In the back of his mind Bud had an idea, but he wasn't ready to propose it yet. He kept in touch, checking in on Craig.

Winter turned to spring, Craig got progressively worse, and still no one could figure out exactly what was wrong with him. There were heart issues, to be sure, but something else was at work. Linda Lewis had all but moved into the hospital, trying her best to keep her husband's spirits up when he was conscious, making friends with the families of other patients who were fighting for their lives, shooing away the chaplain because, she said, he made her nervous.

No one told her that her husband was probably a terminal case. Craig didn't have a shot at a transplant: when doctors finally biopsied his heart tissue, they discovered amyloidosis, a disease in which proteins form toxic sheets in the organs of the body, eventually destroying them from within. Amyloidosis was extremely rare—the last case any doctor in Houston had seen was five years earlier—and it moved through the body with lethal speed. Trying to buy time, Bud implanted a different pump, called a TandemHeart, as a stopgap, but time was running out. Five days was the usual limit someone could survive with such a device.

By the beginning of March, Craig had been on the Tandem-Heart for fourteen days, and Bud figured that even if everything went right, he had, at best, twelve more to live.

Whenever Bud saw Linda, he recognized the look in her eyes. He had seen it as a med student, as an intern, and as a flight surgeon in

Vietnam—that silent plea for the impossible. It was a lonely place, being the last person standing between life and death; sometimes he could help, and sometimes he couldn't. Even after decades as a surgeon, Bud still saw mystery in the patients he saved and the patients he lost: the question wasn't why people died, he liked to say, but why they lived. Medicine had been practiced since the beginnings of man; medical libraries overflowed with tome after tome that attempted to keep pace with the ever-expanding rate of medical knowledge. Bud himself had spent more than fifty years at patients' bedsides. But with all his knowledge, he couldn't predict who would make it and who would not, and there had been plenty of times when he just ran out of things to offer. Linda's look was the reason Bud had spent the better part of his life trying to come up with ways to help patients with sick hearts; he had never been able to tolerate the sense of helplessness that came over him when he couldn't pull off a save.

Now the only thing Bud had to offer Craig and Linda Lewis was a big risk—or, from the view of a dying man, not much risk at all. Late one night, Bud put in a call to Linda. "If we could just get in front of the amyloidosis," he told her, "maybe we could buy you some more time." A few days, weeks, he just didn't know. Then he began explaining to her, as best he could, something new he had been working on for several years with another surgeon: an artificial heart. They had tested this new device in animals and it had worked fine. But he had to be honest: he didn't know whether it would work in humans, and if it did, for how long. They would be taking a big chance that would probably benefit more people in the future than her husband today.

Linda listened quietly, without interruption, but spoke as soon as Bud was done. "Craig's gonna want a manual," she said.

THE WIZARD, 2015

Bud Frazier sometimes wandered through St. Luke's Hospital like a large wraith in a white coat. For decades he had traveled from his office in the Texas Heart Institute through the maze of attached hallways that was St. Luke's, a worn paperback perpetually open in his hand, often something by Shakespeare, rarely anything that could remotely be considered popular. At seventy-five, Bud had earned certain privileges: The right to walk and read, which kept a lot of people out of his way. The right to leave towels in swirls and eddies on the floor of the private bathroom in his office. The right to check his cellphone at society galas, because people assumed he was checking on patients, and sometimes he was. A few years back, Bud had had to give up his black cowboy boots for running shoes, because surgery, especially lengthy surgeries, could be as hard on your legs and your back as it was on your hands. He'd had two brand-new titanium knees put in last summer and had been glad when he was able to give up the fancy cane he'd had to use. It made pretty women solicitous, which made him grouchy.

Bud's wife, Rachel, liked to describe her husband, generously, as an absentminded professor, but like many people at the top of their fields, Bud had lots of folks looking after the mundane details of his life so that he could focus on his work. He often forgot his wallet; he did not balance his checkbook; he did not "do" email. Once, when he could not find a parking place for a gala, he parked his old Jaguar—a gift from a grateful patient—on the front patio of the Houston Museum of Natural Science, barely missing the fountains. Everyone forgave him his trespasses: Bud could list, among a very long list of friends and associates and patients and their family members, everyone from Mehmet Oz to the memoirist Mary Karr, from Dick Cheney to Bono, from Olivia de Havilland to various Middle Eastern and European royalty. He had a long-suffering assistant named Libby Schwenke who was charged with getting him from point A to point B, whether it was from Houston to Kazakhstan or just across the Texas Medical Center, which, unfortunately for her, was the largest in the world. Even so, Bud was perennially late, famous for slipping into a party or a lecture long after it was in progress, which allowed him to be simultaneously unobtrusive and a center of attention. Time for Bud was negotiable after so many years operating on the very sick, who didn't follow schedules either.

So here he was, at the crack of dawn, alone. Docs a lot younger than Bud, with better knees but slower hands, were still at home next to their sleeping wives at five-thirty in the morning. Whether he could admit it or not, Bud preferred his office to his home, surrounded by the books that were always in danger of tumbling off the shelves—valuable first editions and ratty paperbacks; Plutarch, Dickens, Dostoyevsky, a few nods to the likes of Hilary Mantel and Larry McMurtry. His literary tastes were a lot more high-minded than those of the average medical student rotating through the Texas Heart Institute, a fact he sometimes couldn't resist noting—to his med students. (When it came to literature, Bud was an equal-opportunity snob: introduced to U2 frontman Bono by a wealthy friend, Bud was appalled when the Irish rock star didn't immediately recognize some lines Bud recited from Yeats.)

Bud opened the door and stepped into the outer office, with the bank of secretarial cubicles on one side and a wall of framed photos and clippings on the other. Because there wasn't any natural light here, the pictures were as fresh as the day they had been taken: photos of Bud with his mentors, Dr. Michael DeBakey and Dr. Denton Cooley, who had been among the most famous heart surgeons of their day in the years from 1960 to 1980 or so. In another photo, Bud posed with Christiaan Barnard, the South African surgeon who had shocked the world—and set off major envy attacks among his colleagues—by performing the first human heart transplant in 1969. There was a photo of Bud with the longest-living heart transplant patient in the world—his patient—and next to it a twenty-year-old story from the *New York Times* about the success of the left ventricular assist device. Bud had an impressive collection of medals, and on the highest shelf above his assistant's desk, a tenuously crowded collection of crystal vases and plaques etched with his name. There was a framed portrait with a quote from Teddy Roosevelt—a favorite of many aggrieved surgeons—about the man in the arena who, "if he fails, fails while daring greatly, so that his place shall never be with those cold and timid souls who neither know victory nor defeat." Close to that was another maxim: "No one gets in to see the Wizard, not nobody, not no how," a former student had written, quoting the *Wizard of Oz*. It was an inside joke. Everyone got in; Bud Frazier was incapable of telling anyone no.

He padded down the dim hallway, past the open door to Billy Cohn's office, the heart surgeon who sometimes helped Bud—who was not mechanically minded—develop devices for ailing hearts. As often happened, Billy wasn't there; he spent weeks in other countries, lecturing on and testing his many inventions. But even when Billy was gone, his office seemed to be fully inhabited by him, by the whirs and clicks of all sorts of tiny machines that entranced him, by the perpetual motion of his screen savers on at least three computers and laptops, by the eerie blue light they projected around the room. Billy hung his oldest prototypes on the walls with regular nails and thumbtacks and sometimes, Scotch tape: a bent fork, a lariat made of thin white tubing, a kitchen spatula—all variants of things he had invented that went into people's bodies or helped heart surgeons do their jobs. Bud's office walls were paneled and book lined. Billy filled his space with trinkets, doodads, and gewgaws that only he fully understood. There were the books on magic piled on top of medical texts and a deck of cards on his desk—Billy performed at national conventions. There was a cover photo from a weekly tabloid of Billy playing the trombone with his band at a bar called the Boondocks, a late-night date he kept every Tuesday. This was a man whose fingers were still only when he was sleeping—if in fact Billy ever slept. Unlike Bud, Billy didn't keep a couch in his office.

Bud left his office suite and made for the elevators. He didn't stop on the ground floor, where he might have taken in his first exposure of the day to natural light—it poured into the three-story atrium of the Heart Institute's Denton A. Cooley wing, as if God himself were blessing the place. Instead, Cooley officed just behind the soaring space; at ninety-two, he still came in every day, getting around the hospital on a scooter or being pushed in a wheelchair by one of his former nurses. Fortunately, he was not such a bad driver.

At an elevator, Bud punched the button for the basement.

In the old days—the sixties, seventies, the early eighties—the animal research lab had been on the third floor of St. Luke's, adjacent to the operating rooms. Such a location would be unethical now—who would even think of it?—but back then laws on animal research were more lax, and, besides, if Cooley wanted it there so he could duck in and out between surgeries, he got whatever he wanted because he'd founded the heart institute for starters, and he brought in the most patients, meaning, of course, he brought in the most money. The biggest problem with that location was that the obstetrics ward was also on the same floor, so the moans of women in labor were accompanied by the sounds of dogs barking, cows mooing, or the screeching of baboons.

The end of that situation came with what Bud still called The Incident of the Yucatan Mini Pigs. He had been working on some experiments that involved welding blood vessels together with lasers, and it turned out the veins of the 100-pound pigs were the closest things to those of humans. But then someone snuck in one night and freed the pigs from their cages—probably an administrator, Bud still speculated darkly—so about twenty of them went racing into the maternity ward. Bud had to round up the mini pigs himself, herding them back into the lab as they snorted and relieved themselves all over the place. Soon after that, Cooley got a new cardiac research lab in the basement.

Bud had been in charge for the last forty years or so.

The door to the lab had a window covered with a venetian blind, a nod to security along with the key card Bud swiped to let himself in. The place wasn't much to look at, which made it camera ready for PETA membership drives. The floor was linoleum, and the tile walls were that sorry shade of prison green. The animals in metal stanchions—like modern-day stocks—raised their heads to look at Bud: one goat, one cow. At his arrival they blinked and chewed the hay at their feet, paying him little mind.

He had told his mother, a schoolteacher, that he'd decided to become a doctor one night while she was cooking him dinner. He was in from Austin and the University of Texas, back home in the small town of Stephenville. She kept stirring a pot on the stove while he explained his choice; she didn't stop to look at him. "Well," she said, when he finished, "I think you should do what you want, but

I never knew you to much like to kill things." Well, "killing things" wasn't his goal as a doctor, but being an attentive son, Bud intuited her meaning: with a mother's impeccable memory, she was referencing that time he was eight years old and his friend Butch Henry had shot a rabbit in the brush. Bud raced to the site and found a mother rabbit dying, her unborn babies tumbling out of her belly where the shotgun pellets had torn her open. Bud gathered up the tiny bundle of kits, raced home and tried to save them, but he was too late.

His life's through line became saving the unsavable. This made Bud not just famous and respected, but beloved, and not just in Houston but anywhere he had taken care of sick people around the world. But he still had one goal to accomplish before he hung it up: Bud wanted to see a working artificial heart become a reality, a total replacement that could be implanted and then forgotten, as his friendly rival, another famous heart surgeon, Robert Jarvik liked to say. And, finally, Bud felt that he was close.

In the next room, Bud found the calf. He was a Corriente, a smallish breed descended from the Spanish. His coat was a reddish brown, soft and thick; in a different life he would have spent his youth avoiding cowboys in a roping competition at a rodeo. Instead, he was standing up in his small stall, wires and tubes running in and out of his chest every which way, hooked up to enough monitors better suited to send him to the moon. Bud scratched the calf's forehead and thought, as he often did, that they were such sweet animals.

Nearby, on a pile of old hospital blankets, was Daniel Timms, PhD, who had been sleeping there all night. A youthful-looking thirty-five-year-old biomedical engineer from Brisbane, Australia, Timms was a slight, tightly wound man with piercing blue eyes and a snaggletooth that, depending on which nurse you asked, made him more or less movie-star handsome. His short brown hair was often tousled, and he always seemed in need of a shave. Daniel wasn't known around the THI for his sense of humor, but the rumors of his genius gave him a pass.

The calf shifted its weight and Daniel's eyes followed, watching the animal's chest move in and out. Then, reflexively, Daniel's eyes moved to the monitor. It registered the calf's vital signs as completely normal.

Or rather, completely normal considering that yesterday, in an eight-hour operation, Drs. Frazier and Cohn had sliced out the calf's heart and replaced it with Daniel Timms' invention, a device smaller than a tennis ball, that, once stitched in place, took over all the functions of a normal heart. Except, that is, for one thing: the calf had no detectable pulse. One small titanium disc spinning in its housing—at four thousand times a minute—was the only thing keeping this calf alive.

HOW HARD COULD IT BE?

Deep in the bowels of the Smithsonian Institution's National Museum of American History is a section of a storeroom with a particular set of drawers. If you go through the proper channels, a friendly curator will let you in and, donning a pair of gloves, open the drawers to reveal some very strange and pretty unappealing-looking devices. Some are made of plastic faded to the color of old chicken broth—though that's a nice way of putting it. Others contain discolored tubes and fabric stained the color of rust, or, more precisely, old blood. Virtually all of them have two parts stuck together and most have large holes on each side, giving them the look of cockeyed binoculars.

They do not look like anything a sane person would want stuck inside him- or herself. But in fact these devices represent what has been, for a very long time, the holy grail of medicine: a dependable artificial heart that works on its own inside the body, just like an artificial hip or knee. The cure for cancer runs a very close second to this pursuit, but the fact is, heart disease kills more people around the world than all cancers combined: 17.9 million people or 32 percent of all deaths in 2015. (Three million women in the

United States had breast cancer last year, while 12 million had heart disease.) And while these numbers are declining in the developed world, about 26 million Americans currently have heart disease; 2,150 of them die of it each *day*, an average of one death every forty seconds, or one out of every six deaths in the United States. The number of people who die from heart attacks may have also fallen significantly over the years, thanks to better care and better technology, but now a greater problem is heart failure, a chronic, progressive illness interrupted with life-threatening crises. The American Heart Association's figures show that 5.7 million people suffered from heart failure in the period from 2009 to 2012, but that number jumped to 6.5 million, a 14 percent increase, from 2012 to 2014. Heart transplants have become the solution of choice for disease that is beyond treatment with diet, lifestyle, and medication, but surgeons and their desperate patients know the truth: in any given year there were only 2,500 hearts available for transplant, with about 50,000 people on the waiting list. In other words, there are twenty times more losers than winners.

Meanwhile, costs are also increasing. The total direct and indirect expense of cardiovascular disease and stroke in the United States was estimated to be $312.6 billion in 2009, a number that includes not just deaths but lost productivity. And the numbers are still rising: the total number of inpatient cardiovascular operations and procedures increased 28 percent between 2000 and 2010, from nearly 6 million to 7.5 million.

If a heart attack or stroke doesn't cause instant death, life still becomes circumscribed in unimaginable ways. Once the heart has trouble pumping, the lungs start working less efficiently, and begin to fill up with fluid. Breathing becomes labored, so the slightest move, from the sofa to a sunny patio, or from bed to the bathroom, might as well be a marathon. Every move causes dizziness and shortness of breath. With circulation reduced, the liver, the kidneys, everything, slows down because of a lack of revivifying blood. The stomach and ankles swell, creating the sensation of walking on a bed of needles. A fog of fatigue sets in and stays. Or, suddenly, the heart races as if frantic to escape the chest. Life could be taken away in an instant; that fear becomes a constant companion, like living with your own ghost. Drugs and surgeries help to a point, but eventually you run out of options and then you will land on a long list for a transplant that will probably never happen.

The person who comes up with a way to replace a failing heart with an artificial one, then, will save countless lives and change the future of humankind, much as Louis Pasteur or Sigmund Freud did, or Jonas Salk or Marie Curie. And, of course, the doctor or engineer (or, more likely, the team) who figures out how to make one will likely become very, very rich. The perks, on the surface at least, look incredibly attractive, which is why inventors around the world are desperately trying to come up with a dependable, implantable artificial heart.

But just as the public is not very open to changing unhealthy habits, it's not very tolerant of mistakes in innovation, especially when lives are at stake. Many modern-day inventors of almost any stripe would probably say that if they had known what they were getting into—the maze of technological, legal, medical, and ethical challenges—they might not have even tried.

There are also the unique questions that have swirled around the creation of the artificial heart since its beginnings more than fifty years ago. Is it ethical to spend millions on the development of a machine that could help comparatively few, when preventive care could help 90 percent of all those who develop heart disease? What would it mean if human life could be extended not just by years but by decades? How much is that worth, not only in dollars but in some undefined and unfathomable emotional currency? What would it mean to be alive but literally heartless?

To explore the workings of the heart is to discover a form and a func
tion that can inspire thoughts of the divine in the most determined
atheist. It is a marvel of strength, efficiency, and tenacity. About the
size of a human fist—your fist, custom-designed to your unique
size—it nestles perfectly at an angle deep inside the chest, protected
by the rib cage and a cushion of lungs. Weighing about eight to ten
ounces, less than a one-pound sack of sugar or a running shoe, it has
four hollow chambers, atria and ventricles that look, in pictures, like
ancient temples carved out of caves. Those hollows hold perfectly
regulated amounts of blood as they pass through on their way to the
body. The heart also has its own system of valves, muscles, and electrical currents that make sure nothing goes wrong. In fact, it's easy
to believe in the heart as a near-perpetual motion machine: it beats
60 to 80 times per minute, about 115,000 times a day, more than
2.5 billion beats in an average lifetime. Someone trying to squeeze
a rubber ball at the same rate would last about a minute or two, yet
the heart keeps pace continuously, whether a person is running a
marathon, making love, arguing with a coworker, or getting a good
night's sleep. The heart is always there, keeping time to life itself.

The heart is actually two pumping systems in one, and the two
sides never meet, a little like trains passing in a station. At the center of this station is one muscle contraction that works a little like
a dispatcher. Blood comes into the heart through two large veins,
depleted of the oxygen it's used for its long journey through the
body's circulatory system. It first arrives in the right atrium, which,
once full, contracts, pushing the blood down into the right ventricle through a one-way valve (imagine a system of locks). Another
contraction pushes the blood that was already occupying that space

through another one-way valve into the pulmonary artery and into the lungs, where oxygen refreshes the blood.

From there, the blood exits through the pulmonary vein back into the heart, this time into the left atrium. This side of the heart is responsible for the hardest work: with each contraction, the muscles here have to be strong enough to send the blood from the left atrium into the left ventricle, and then into the main artery, the aorta, and out into the body. In a healthy person, the heart pumps about two thousand gallons of blood a day for this trip. That's six or so quarts, or a little more than five and a half liters* in medspeak, a minute.

Like a home, the heart has an electrical system in addition to its plumbing system of pipes and pumps: the heart contracts thanks to an invisible current that stops and starts. In between, it rests. This contraction and release—systole and diastole to professionals—is, of course, the heartbeat or pulse, the phenomenon known to virtually everyone on earth as the *lub-dub* sound that tells us we are alive.

That's how things work when all goes well. If there's a problem with the electrical system, the heart can stop abruptly, like a car with a dead motor. A worn-out artery can rupture like an old garden hose. If the heart muscle is not strong enough to push blood out into the body, clots in the pooling blood block arterial passages and cause strokes. A heart the size of a basketball might sound like a very strong organ, but in fact it's a sign that the muscles of the organ have had to grow larger and larger just to keep a weak system pumping.

Most cardiac surgeons approach these problems with all the romance and sentimentality of an oil field worker confronting a leaky pipeline. The heart is just a pump, they will tell you, usually with a shrug—a statement that actually tells you a lot more about heart

---

* Since liters are the standard measurement in medicine, I have used them throughout this book. One quart is equal to .95 liters.

surgeons than the heart. These are physicians who have less in common with your kindhearted family doctor than with the first people who crossed Everest's Khumbu Icefall or took the first steps on the moon. Medical explorers, like all explorers, tend to be brilliant, obsessive, brave, and arrogant; many of them were and are ill-suited to societal norms, craving adulation while, at the same time, behaving in ways that don't exactly build affection. Maybe they have to be all those things: you don't really want the person who cuts into your heart to lack self-confidence.

If the heart is truly simple and reducible, something challenging but ultimately conquerable . . . well, maybe minimizing its power is the only way we could have gotten where we are today. Bud Frazier likes to say that practicing medicine satisfies needs that are more metaphysical, for both doctors and their patients: "It's something we do, like art or music," he says. "Every primitive tribe has a Medicine Man," meaning that in every era humanity wants to believe in its healers, who might be nothing more than salesmen with a good line.

Heart disease is, in fact, a fairly modern phenomenon. Throughout most of history, people didn't live long enough to die of it, though it has been found in Egyptian mummies—nature's revenge, maybe, for royal Egyptians who ate too much rich food. Most people died from other causes, including war, famine, and plagues, until fairly recently. One reason our understanding of the heart progressed slowly is that for centuries the idea of cutting open a body and actually touching the heart was seen as an act against God. The heart was not "just a pump" then—it was the seat of the soul. "For where your treasure is, there your heart will be also," says Matthew 6:21; or, to take a sample from Shakespeare's *Hamlet*: "Give me that man / That is not passion's slave, and I will wear him / In my heart's core, ay, in my heart of heart."

As late as 1900, the leading cause of death was pneumonia. All the way through the first half of the twentieth century, people died of things like the flu, pneumonia, and tuberculosis, and medical researchers frantically searched for drugs that cured infectious diseases. When they succeeded, greater numbers of people started living much longer lives. But then the medical profession had a new, mysterious epidemic to contend with. People—especially middle-aged white men—began dropping dead at astounding rates from something that was soon called a heart "attack." So swift was the rise of this new blight that it was already killing more people than TB, pneumonia, kidney disease, or cancer. The symptoms were hard to detect, because, as one doctor wrote during the Depression era, "There is not a single sensation associated with real heart disease which may not be caused by some other, and often insignificant disorder." Physicians weren't necessarily wrong to insist that avoiding infection, "as from the mouth and tonsils," was one way to prevent heart disease, but they didn't have many ideas beyond that. And if a heart problem happened to be diagnosed before it was fatal, there wasn't much to be done: bed rest—six or so months at the least—was pretty much all they had to offer.

Then, on September 24, 1955, President Dwight D. Eisenhower was enjoying a much-needed vacation in Denver. He loved nothing more than a good game of golf, and that afternoon he was playing at the cushy Cherry Hills Golf Course. But he was the president, and interruptions then could not be easily dispatched with an iPhone. Eisenhower had to keep returning to the clubhouse to take calls from his Secretary of State, John Foster Dulles. By the fourth interruption, Eisenhower was so angry about the disruptions that, according to one writer, "the veins stood out on his forehead like whipcords." At around the same time, his stomach started bothering him. Eisenhower thought it was just indigestion—after all, he had eaten a burger with a slice of Bermuda onion for lunch. But later that night, he woke up with a crushing pain in his chest. His wife, Mamie, had the good sense to call his personal physician, who dashed to the president's bedside at 2:00 a.m.

Depending on which account you believe, he may or may not have misdiagnosed Eisenhower's condition. Over the next few days, the president was examined by army doctors, and then civilian doctors. There wasn't much debate about the diagnosis at that point: Eisenhower had had a heart attack. "I had the unpleasant fact that I was indeed a sick man," he would later write in his memoirs.

The illnesses of Woodrow Wilson and Franklin Roosevelt were never made public. Eisenhower's heart attack changed that custom, though when his condition was made public, aides played down its seriousness, fearing for his reelection prospects and his power on the world stage. Indeed, the next Monday, the Dow Jones dropped by 6 percent, a loss that came out to about $14 billion and was the biggest since the 1929 crash. The head of what was then the nascent National Heart Institute tried to calm things down by declaring that at least half a dozen members of Congress had sufficiently recovered from heart problems to return to work, including Texas senator Lyndon Baines Johnson.

There was a lot of very public speculation over what might have caused Eisenhower's heart attack, including his age and sex, heredity, and "an ambitious personality." His high-altitude golf game came up, and so did drinking alcohol, "local religious and social customs," and smoking. The president was a lifelong smoker, up to four packs a day. But the curious thing was, Eisenhower didn't need to spend the usual six months in bed to recover from his heart attack. And he really didn't want to. He was up and about in several days, and it was a matter of a few weeks before he was back at the office. Any thoughts that he would not be able to run for reelection were promptly dismissed. In fact, as Eisenhower's health improved, both his doctors and his operatives proved themselves masters of the newish art of spin. One doctor reported, for instance, that Eisenhower had had a "successful bowel movement," believing such news would reassure educated physicians around the country that he was on the mend.

And he was. Eisenhower finished his second term, though there were a few more health-related cliff-hangers, most of which, in an interesting turnabout, were kept secret. By some estimates, he suffered a stroke and four more heart attacks. When he died in 1969, the cause was said to be congestive heart failure. But the fact that he did recover from the first attack well enough to return to work and win reelection suggested that, maybe, the conventional treatment for heart disease was, in a word, wrong.

THE MAKING OF A SURGEON

When Bud was a kid in the 1940s and 1950s, Paul "Bear" Bryant, who would become nationally famous as head coach of the University of Alabama football team, spent some time as the coach of the Aggies, at Texas A&M. The winningest coach in football history began his tenure there in 1954 by hosting a ten-day "summer camp" in the tiny town of Junction, 240 miles away.

Junction, on the northwestern edge of the Texas Hill Country, has its merits—two lovely, limestone-lined rivers converge there—but few are obvious in the August heat, which was when Bryant set up his training camp. That year, the community was also experiencing the worst drought in recorded history, along with a heat wave that had temperatures hitting 100 degrees almost every day. Despite that, Bryant ran his boys from dawn until 11:00 p.m. He didn't allow water breaks. Offensive players got one towel soaked in cold water to share, defense got the other. In the context of Texas football, especially small-town Texas football, Bryant's techniques were seen as nothing short of brilliant. You had to be tough to win, after all, and winning at Texas football was about the only thing there was. It didn't matter if you were smart, good-looking, or your daddy owned the bank. If you couldn't stop some two-hundred-pound sixteen-year-old churning toward you on the field, or if you couldn't throw a long pass without some pimply-faced knucklehead from the next town over intercepting, you'd get your ass handed to you by the whole damn town. The coach wanted laps when it was 105 degrees in the shade? Called you a goddamned idiot and threatened to bench your sorry ass for the remainder of the season? You did what you were told, or killed yourself trying. Maybe you hadn't read Darwin in high school, but if you played Texas football, you didn't have to.

In one sense, Bud Frazier was lucky: he was a big kid with natural talent. If he hadn't been, his life would have been hell, because he liked nothing more in the world than reading books—the kiss of death just about everywhere in Texas in those days, but particularly in his hometown of Stephenville, a small town about one hundred empty, arid miles southwest of Fort Worth. Both Bud's parents were teachers—Bud's father had missed the first three years of his son's life while fighting in World War II; he returned quiet and easygoing, if distant, and took a job as a chemistry teacher and coach at a local junior college. His mother, who was far more demanding—at eighty-one she was still correcting Bud's grammar—taught high school English. With neither parent around during the day, Bud and his older sister Marilyn grew up in the care of his maternal grandmother, who taught him to read before he was four. There were also frequent drop-ins from his uncle Mule, whose tall tales of West Texas would forever shape Bud's love of narrative. As Bud grew up, he spent his spare time—and there was a lot of it in Stephenville—consuming everything from *Classics Illustrated* comic books to *Hamlet* (he liked the swordfights but found the love scenes dull). "I read a lot because I hardly ever went to class," he recalled. "I knew if I would feign illness enough my mother would just give up."

Bud was also an absentminded child—his mother wrote lists on his hand with a ballpoint pen when she sent him to the store, so he couldn't lose her instructions—but thanks to her sharpness also became a shrewd assessor of things. He knew, for example, that he had to win fights to protect his reputation, and so he fought, and won most of the time. It would become a point of pride that his grand-father's cousin and namesake had been a mean, ornery gunfighter in the Rio Grande Valley. He passed on dubious bits of wisdom to Bud like "It's hard to kill someone with a knife, you just gotta shoot 'em, that's it." For balance, Bud's great-grandfather on his mother's side had been a sheriff. "He killed a number of villains and one Mormon," Bud explained.

Stephenville was not a hotbed of liberalism. No one in town was surprised when the Baptist minister smashed a "sinful" pinball machine with an ax, its death sentence determined by the racy kick of a mechanical cheerleader attached to the flippers. But it was one of the several incidents that indicated to Bud that his days in his hometown were numbered. A football scholarship got him to the University of Texas in 1960, with big plans to play for the legendary Darrell Royal. Then he tore a hamstring first semester, and ended up a history major. Bud embraced big ideas as only a person from a small world can. On an early date with a pretty redhead from Houston, he spent a long time—maybe a very long time—discussing the nature of infinity.

In truth, he had no idea what he wanted to do with his life. He made excellent grades without really trying—Bud was the kind of student who could usually cram for a test the night before and ace it, partly because he had something of a photographic memory. He thought about becoming a Methodist minister, and then maybe a dentist, or a lawyer, or a teacher, and then dismissed them all. "I just wanted something that didn't require me to lie, cheat, or steal," he would say. "And I didn't know anything about the world as a twenty-one-year-old." He was reading a lot of Chekhov at the time and liked the author's descriptions of doctors' lives. That's how Bud decided on a medical career.

He hadn't taken any undergrad pre-med courses but managed, once he put his mind to it, to finish all the required work in a year. Then, without much more thought, he decided on Baylor College of Medicine, not because it was then one of the best programs in the country but because it was in Houston. The redhead who had listened so patiently to his soliloquy on infinity was now living there. Her name was Rachel, and he was in love with her.

—◦◦◦—

Michael DeBakey had landed in Houston about twenty years earlier, in 1948. The city had around half a million people, some of whom had far more money and ambition than clear-eyed direction—at least beyond the notion to be, somehow, "great." The largest city in Texas, Houston was home to the nation's swiftly growing oil business, which was fueling the booming postwar economy. Smoke from the refineries smudged the sky above the south end of town, while the port of Houston, already the second-largest in the country, was clogged with tankers ferrying petrochemicals all over the world. Tudor-style mansions the size of small castles lined the leafy streets of neighborhoods like River Oaks and Shadyside. If some of the civic leaders were in the mold of Edna Ferber's crass, shrewd Jett Rink, other prominent Houstonians were fiercely determined to create a modern, sophisticated city out of . . . not much. Partly by design and partly by accident, they created a place that was less hidebound and more open to opportunity—at least for white men—than any other in the United States. In Houston, success mattered; family pedigree or a high-toned college education did not. The oilman's optimism set the tone: failure was just an unlucky bump on the road to getting really, really rich. It was also important that Houston was seen to be going places, instead of being just another hick Texas town. The city was ripe for a man with dreams and ambitions the size of DeBakey's.

It wasn't a perfect fit. DeBakey was from Lake Charles, Louisiana, the favored son of Lebanese Christian immigrants who had prospered there. Houston was not very diverse back then—minorities mostly consisted of blacks and Hispanics—and the ruling class tended to be white and members of the Baptist or Methodist church. De-Bakey was small in stature, highly educated, and quite worldly. He sported a tiny, fussy mustache. At the time of his arrival in Houston, he somewhat resembled a Vichy-regime villain in a World War II movie. There was nothing of the down-home, never-met-a-stranger veneer Texans in general and Houstonians in particular so valued. DeBakey had his charms, but he applied them mostly to those who could help him accomplish his goals.

He was nothing if not focused. DeBakey's parents believed him to be a genius, and he didn't question their assessment: valedictorian of his high school class, he finished college at Tulane after just two years. Still, it is possible to believe that being the smartest, littlest, and, maybe, oddest kid in your elementary school wasn't easy. He read the encyclopedia; he played the saxophone; he grew vegetables in his father's garden. This was the American South. "Mike got beat up on his way to school and on his way home," a friend told *Life* magazine. Some kids would have been defeated. DeBakey was galvanized.

He stayed at Tulane to get his medical degree and at twenty-three became responsible for one medical advance: he adapted an older device called a roller pump for use in an early version of the heart-lung machine, a crucial invention that decades later would keep patients alive during cardiovascular surgery. He finished his internship and residency in the bedlam that was New Orleans' infamous Charity Hospital, where he became the protégé of one of the South's most prominent physicians, Alton Ochsner. Ochsner's motto was "early to bed, early to rise, work hard, and publicize"—a maxim DeBakey would take to heart.

At just twenty-seven, with his father's financial backing, De-Bakey headed to prestigious surgical fellowships in Strasbourg and at the University of Heidelberg, further distinguishing himself from run-of-the-mill American doctors. He then returned to Tulane, where he joined the surgical faculty. It was there that some of his most distinctive characteristics became apparent. While DeBakey's colleagues admired his skills in the operating room, he earned the nickname "Black Mike" because he was so imperious. Ochsner was always quick to forgive his interns a mishap or two—he was given to teachable moments—but DeBakey could never let go of the slightest infraction. He made scenes, embarrassed underlings in public for tiny errors, and fired residents on the spot for even less. Yes, a mistake in surgery could mean the difference between life and death, but some errors—like interrupting DeBakey when he was deep in thought—did not seem to warrant exile from the Tulane garden. Except to DeBakey.

On the other hand, DeBakey's decisiveness served him well when he left New Orleans to join the military in 1942. He secured a job as a member of the Surgical Consultants Division in the Office of the Surgeon General of the Army, and by 1945 was the director. DeBakey proved himself a relentless and visionary master of organization. Seeing too many soldiers dying on battlefields, he helped create the first mobile army surgical hospitals, for which he received the prestigious Legion of Merit. He lobbied tenaciously for better medical care for veterans, especially improvements in what was then known as the Veterans Administration hospital system, and for increased medical research, seeing in this new patient pool an opportunity to improve public health on a wider scale. During his years in the military, DeBakey also became a master of strategy, tactics, and politics; he was expert at managing his superiors and dictating to (sometimes terrorizing) subordinates. He was fearless in the face of opposition when he knew he was right, and in DeBakey's mind, he was always right.

Prominent Houstonians had started building the Texas Medical Center in 1943. Over the next few years, they used their wealth to supplement the best hospital, Hermann, with a cancer hospital, a navy hospital, and a limestone-faced main building for a medical school—Baylor College of Medicine, which had spent its first Houston years in a repurposed Sears Roebuck store. The medical center, such as it was then, sat on the edge of a large city park at the south end of town. Deer still grazed there, sometimes serving as dinner for urban hunters.

The board had a grand vision: to build the biggest and best medical center in the world. (This was Texas, after all.) To achieve this goal, the members needed a leader who could make this happen out of little more than thin air. It wasn't long before they set their sights on DeBakey, who after the war was back at Tulane as the chief of surgery. But DeBakey wasn't interested. He toured what passed for the Baylor campus and then wrote a three-page letter explaining why he could not possibly take the job. Baylor, he wrote, was a "third-rate" medical school. It had no full-time faculty. General practitioners taught surgery because Baylor had no board-certified surgeons. Even worse, Baylor had no affiliated hospitals where students could get hands-on training. And so on.

Ochsner urged DeBakey to reconsider. "They have big plans and they don't have anybody there that knows what the Hell to do," he told his protégé. Besides, DeBakey could always come back to Tulane if things didn't work out.

And so in 1948 he went, with his young wife, Diana. DeBakey's father bought the young couple an impressive white Tudorish mansionette on Cherokee, a locale that was a short walk down oak-lined Main Street to Baylor. Dr. DeBakey did not like being too far from his patients.

He wasn't met with open arms. Houston's established physicians were not an open-minded, generous lot, and they resented DeBakey from the start. They had no intention of sending him any of *their* patients for *his* surgical practice. He was arrogant, they said. He wasn't nice. He talked to them like they were children. DeBakey quit at least once, abandoning the med center to work in a decrepit hospital downtown, determined to build his reputation on his own. Eventually, however, he was lured back to Baylor—with more money and more power, including the title of chief of surgery. Even though no one asked outright, DeBakey accepted the charge of transforming Baylor into one of the country's best medical schools, and the Texas Medical Center into the largest in the world.

It was a good time for ambitious plans. John F. Kennedy defeated Richard Nixon in 1960. Just forty-three, he was the youngest president elected in American history. If, in retrospect, the success of Kennedy's brief tenure—a thousand days before his assassination in November 1963—is subject to debate, no one can argue the inspirational power he had over the American people. Eisenhower may have been part of a generation that led the United States to victory in World War II, but JFK, young and startlingly handsome, Harvard-educated, sophisticated, and possessed of great wit, made Americans, especially young Americans, feel that anything was possible.

That was never truer than on a hot, sunny day, September 12, 1962, when the president spoke to an exultant Houston crowd of

35,000 at the enormous Rice University stadium in Houston, Texas, thirty miles or so from the headquarters of the four-year-old National Aeronautics and Space Administration. The location was not coincidental. Nor was it coincidental that the United States was scrambling to keep up with the Soviet Union in the race to conquer outer space.

Leaning into the lectern, JFK made a passionate pledge that was a clarion call for a new era: the United States would put a man on the moon within the next eight years. "We choose to go to the moon in this decade and do the other things, not because they are easy, but because they are hard," the president said. "Because that goal will serve to organize and measure the best of our energies and skills, because that challenge is one that we are willing to accept, one we are unwilling to postpone, and one which we intend to win."

It was against this backdrop—a national hunger for new ideas, for innovation, for new global power—that eight months later, in May 1963, Dr. Michael DeBakey made an appearance before the Senate Committee on Health in Washington, DC. No one could argue that, on first sight, he shared JFK's charisma. He was fifty-five; small and slight, he wore thick, horn-rimmed glasses and his dark, coarse hair was brushed back from his receding hairline. He had a nose a toucan would envy. But DeBakey, like JFK, had a gift for oratory and persuasion. And he had passion to spare.

He sat confidently before a group of rapt senators, many of whom he knew by name, many of whom he had treated, or he had treated their wives or fathers or uncles or some other great-aunt's second cousin twice removed. DeBakey remembered them by name too—all of them. He was introduced as the professor and chairman of Baylor's Department of Surgery and as a former member of the National Heart Institute Advisory Council, but DeBakey was by then much more: he was arguably the most famous heart surgeon in the world, a nationally renowned adviser whose opinion was sought on everything from the design of heart valves to public health to the vicissitudes of Washington politics. He advised senators and the president on countless medical issues, including the dangers of smoking long before others would concur.

In the process, the self-made surgeon from Lake Charles now had a vast, ever-expanding network of contacts to Get Things Done. The Houston oilmen who had helped fund Baylor introduced De-Bakey to their pals in Congress and the White House; DeBakey's fellow officers from his wartime years—he had achieved the rank of colonel—were now dispersed around the country, most of them in positions of power as well. DeBakey was also a winner of the Lasker Award in 1963, American medicine's most prestigious prize, given to physicians who made outstanding advances in clinical medical research.

Winning the Lasker Prize was not entirely coincidental. DeBakey had become a crucial member of philanthropist Mary Lasker's circle. Lasker was a Radcliffe-educated powerhouse whose second husband, Albert, owned an ad agency that at one time had the job of getting more women to smoke cigarettes. Soon enough, though, the pair changed course and created a substantial fund to support medical research. By the time of Albert's death in 1950, Mary had organized a group of high-minded and politically savvy operators determined to make the US government improve the health of its people. In the process, Lasker and her cohorts became experts at the kind of public relations–driven, pay-to-play lobbying that exists today. DeBakey and Sidney Farber, the Nobel Prize–winning cancer researcher from Harvard, were Lasker's go-to experts when she needed a physician to browbeat government officials and marshal public opinion; in particular, when she needed someone to explain why the money appropriated for medical research just wasn't enough. At this, Lasker and her cohorts were extraordinarily successful: the budget for the

National Institutes of Health went from $460 million between 1946 and 1961 to $1 billion five or so years later.

Attitudes had changed since the US victory over the Axis forces in 1945. The economy was strong and growing. The American triumph in World War II had validated our greatness. Science had not only helped to win the war with the deadly success of the Manhattan Project but also saved us from humiliation in the Cold War–dominated space race. Yes, Russian Yuri Gagarin was the first person to orbit the earth in 1961, but after a few false starts astronaut John Glenn caught up in 1962, and made the journey around the world *two more times.* So why couldn't Americans cure cancer and heart disease? And why shouldn't the federal government pay for the research?

—◊◊◊—

The question wasn't rhetorical for Michael DeBakey. He had zeroed in on heart disease as his life's work. Trained as a general surgeon—there wasn't any heart surgery when he was studying medicine—he saw that now the biggest rewards lay in uncovering its mysteries.

He had some stiff competition. During the early twentieth century, heart disease research was the siren's song for ambitious men of medicine. Technological and medical discoveries that would change its detection and treatment followed with breathtaking swiftness. In 1929, a German named Werner Forssman proved it was possible to X-ray the heart by inserting a catheter filled with dye through the veins and directly into the heart—what would come to be known as the common practice of cardiac catheterization. (He was fired for trying it on himself.)

Even so, operating on the heart itself was still inconceivable. No one had any idea how to keep a patient alive and breathing while a surgeon cut into the organ. Then, in 1937, John Gibbon began experimenting with a machine that would keep the heart and lungs operating during surgery, an accomplishment that Leo Eloesser would describe in *Milestones in Chest Surgery* as "among the boldest and the most successful feats of a man's mind." Within two decades, it would become possible to operate on the heart and lungs of a human being without killing him—as long as you could get in and out really, really fast. Too much time "on the pump" created new sets of problems, the worst being that sometimes doctors couldn't wean a patient off of it.

While Gibbon was at work on his machine, a surgeon named Robert E. Gross operated for the first time on the heart of a child, to correct a congenital defect. In 1949, the first portable heart monitor was put to use; the first pacemaker followed a year later, and two years after that, in 1952, the first artificial heart valves were implanted.

But the most important advances of that time were achieved by a dashing Minnesota surgeon by the name of C. Walton Lillehei. In 1952, he performed the first surgical repair of the heart, using a new technique, hypothermia—lowering a patient's body temperature to the point where he was barely alive. Lillehei would go on to become the most influential heart surgeon of the next decade or so, not just for his innovations but because he was a person who made it hard to tell where boldness ended and recklessness began.

Lillehei created a technique called cross circulation that from today's perspective sounds, at best, dicey: he figured out a way to connect the bloodstream of a child to that of his parent during surgery in order to keep blood moving through a young patient's body while he operated. (The joke at the time was that Lillehei had come up with a surgery that had a 200 percent mortality rate.) By 1955, he had abandoned that procedure in favor of his own version of a heart-lung machine. The list of accomplishments goes on: he was the first surgeon to try what would become a pacemaker, and also trained Norman Shumway and Christiaan Barnard, who would go on to become pioneers in heart transplants.

In the race to cure heart disease, however, Michael DeBakey wasn't about to be left behind. As early as 1939, he and Ochsner believed in the dangers of smoking, not just as a contributor to or cause of cancer, but to heart disease too. DeBakey also found a way to use a common synthetic fabric, Dacron, as a replacement for blood vessels in the late 1950s. The story was that he went downtown to Houston's major department store, Foley's, to buy his usual graft material—nylon—but they were out. A salesperson suggested the substitution of something called Dacron. DeBakey went back to the operating room and found that—yes!—the material made stronger and better blood vessels than what he'd been using. Soon enough, the Dacron graft became the standard and DeBakey got the credit. Never one to miss an opportunity to further burnish his reputation, he restaged his discovery for a widely distributed photograph.

Not coincidentally, DeBakey also became a pioneer in the filming of surgeries, usually starring . . . himself. People had a right to see what he was doing, he insisted, when criticized for being a publicity hound. He was also a publishing dervish, thanks largely to two unmarried sisters, Selma and Lois, who followed their older brother from Louisiana to Houston just to help him draft, edit, and submit his ever-growing oeuvre to medical journals. DeBakey was the first surgeon with his own in-house PR firm.

So by the time DeBakey made his pitch to Congress in 1962, he had aligned his ambitions with two crucial items in the healthcare budget. First, he agreed that the National Institutes of Health should fund coronary research centers around the United States. In fact, he had the perfect spot: Baylor College of Medicine. The second was a lot grander: Michael DeBakey wanted money to create nothing less than an artificial heart. If that idea struck many as one straight out of a sci-fi comic book, DeBakey was not among them. He was convinced that the idea of building a heart from scratch was not only possible, but perfectly reasonable.

As DeBakey explained in his silky but authoritative Lake Charles drawl: "We are on the brink today of relieving mankind of its most painful and debilitating afflictions. . . . Surely this is not the time to sit back and be satisfied merely to consolidate our gains or to level off our support of these endeavors." The National Institutes of Health, he said, had "brought American medicine to the forefront of the world. It would be a crime against humanity were we to negate what has been done by proceeding faintheartedly and lacking resolution and the courage of our convictions."

His pitch worked. Congress voted to expand the NIH budget—from $134 million to $215 million. And they granted permission for a special committee to study the feasibility of the artificial heart—with DeBakey as a member, of course. More important for DeBakey, Baylor College of Medicine was one of several institutions given $10 million in federal funds—about $75 million today—to set up a research facility specifically designed to pursue the development of the artificial heart.

DeBakey knew he could make a device that could change the course of history. After all, the heart was just a pump.

—\/\/\—

Even when Bud was a much older and more accomplished man, he could still find himself obsessing about DeBakey. He studied biographies of Joseph Stalin, which offered helpful insights. He gave De-

Bakey his due—a person couldn't have built Baylor and Methodist Hospital, much less the Texas Medical Center, into the globally recognized institutions they had become without an indomitable will. Thanks to DeBakey, Bud and his fellow students had endured the toughest, most challenging program of its day. You were the best, like the Marines. So Bud would never say something as mundane as "That guy was an asshole." Instead, he just told stories.

Bud was twenty-three when he started at Baylor in 1963. DeBakey was as selective of his students as he had been in picking the faculty and staff, which came from the likes of Harvard and Johns Hopkins. There were only seventy-five in each class, and they came not just from Texas colleges and universities but from the best schools across the country: Duke, Pomona, Princeton, Stanford. "Everybody in my class wanted to be either a surgeon or an internist," Bud recalled. "We had one guy that wanted to be an ophthalmologist, but he always had to explain himself when he said he was going to be an ophthalmologist, because that wasn't a real doctor."

Bud figured he would try surgery. He had a lab partner who developed a tremor in his hands, and so Bud ended up doing all the operating for both of them. Within a few weeks, he knew he had found his calling. While others struggled, he knew, in some deep-seated, intuitive way, that he could do it. It wasn't just that his hands were good, or that he had near-perfect recall for the body's anatomy, or that he wasn't afraid when he picked up a scalpel. Bud was like a novelist who understood his story without seeing it on the page; he just knew where he was supposed to go.

Like all Baylor students, he quickly learned that his chief was a mixed blessing. It was best to steer clear of DeBakey as much as possible; only the clueless or heedlessly ambitious asked him questions. You were never supposed to interrupt DeBakey's ostensibly brilliant train of thought. When DeBakey drove his white Maserati to the doors of Baylor at the 5:00 a.m. start of his workday, he wore custom-made royal-blue scrubs; interns waited anxiously to park his car. Greeting him with a sunny "Good morning" was a risk few took. Riding with him to nearby hospitals could be a career ender. God forbid if you pushed an elevator button that slowed his progress when he was on it.

Baylor docs in training were zombies a lot of the time: once De-Bakey's students started working with real patients in their third year, they were expected to take call every other night—to be in the hospital all night and all the next day, while still responding competently to any emergency. It was a lot like combat, which, given DeBakey's military experience, made—some—sense.

On the other hand, DeBakey wasn't around that much, because he was so often off in DC to lobby for something, or in Europe teaching other surgeons some new technique or checking up on a former patient like the Duke of Windsor.

When he was in Houston, DeBakey was a regular if unpredictable presence in his small but active cardiovascular lab, located in the original Baylor building in what was then called the hospital's "Jewish Wing," because it existed thanks to the largesse of Houston's wealthiest Jewish donors. As with so many things DeBakey created, it was devoted to excellence, but the high quality was maintained by a group of people who were, well, odd. A medical degree—or any medical training—was not a requirement, partly because there were no hospital committees then governing medical school labs, partly because DeBakey ran the place, and partly because that was how things went in Houston.

The most valued member of the team may have been a brilliant machinist from New York City by the name of Louis Feldman, a sweet, soft-spoken immigrant originally from Eastern Europe. He and DeBakey were devoted to each other because the self-taught Feldman could fabricate anything DeBakey requested, and that was not easy. There were two black assistants named MC and Fred—their last names have been lost—who performed most of the animal surgery. There was a heart valve expert by the name of William C. Hall, from the University of Kansas, who loved nothing more than making and baking molds for artificial heart parts in his kitchen at home on weekends. Another key staff member was Domingo Liotta, an Argentine surgeon who was both florid and brooding, but like Hall obsessed with the creation of artificial organs. DeBakey had enticed Liotta to Houston from the employ of Willem Kolff at the prestigious Cleveland Clinic, a coup at the time because, for people who followed such things, Kolff was considered the father of the artificial organ field. A Dutchman who fought in the resistance during the war, he'd gone on to invent the first dialysis machine—an artificial kidney. With various associates, Kolff had begun implanting prototypes for an artificial heart in dogs in the 1950s; one lived for what was then the miraculous period of nine hours.

There was also an assortment of interns and medical students rotating in and out, not the least among them a tall, goofy country boy who went by the name of Bud.

Looking back, Bud figured that he was able to survive his sentence with DeBakey for two reasons: the prior abuse he had put up with from his football coaches, and the good manners his parents had stressed. They had taught him to keep his head down, work hard, and (mostly) respect his elders. Bud quickly understood, for instance, the dangers of asking DeBakey any questions, so he didn't. Baylor's motto was "see one, do one, teach one," which from today's perspective sounds like a recipe for a lawsuit. It worked well at the time because there was (a) less to learn and (b) the punishment for slipping up in even the smallest ways got you fired. DeBakey made experienced residents stand in the corner when they displeased him in the operating room. He fired a nurse who was just a week away from her retirement when she was too slow following orders.

When Bud slipped up—and everyone did—he braced for the public shaming. The smooth Louisiana inflection DeBakey used in normal discourse—such as there was—would become a hiss, and the list of sins could go on for what seemed like an eternity. Once, Bud got the time wrong for a procedure and ran late. "Of course, if you *cared,* you would have been there *early,*" Bud would recall, in an admirable imitation of DeBakey's voice, and with the same accuracy with which he recited Shakespearean sonnets. "If you *cared,* you would have had to learn something. But of course, to do that, you'd have to *care.* But obviously you didn't *care* . . ." and so on. Other times, DeBakey would just cut to the chase with the favorite, "You're either stupid or you don't care." Often, DeBakey added a punch to the chest with one of his strong, bony knuckles. Anger management training had not yet come into being.

Bud took cover under the tutelage of another Baylor surgeon named Stanley Crawford. Crawford was a stocky, soft-spoken Alabaman, who had come to Baylor from Harvard Medical School and Massachusetts General Hospital. His expertise was heart disease and heart surgery, but he loved nothing more than operating on weekends in the small suburban hospitals ringing Houston, oil refinery towns with deceptively pretty names like Baytown and Deer Park. The patients were mostly blue-collar workers and their families—Houston was a blue-collar town then—people of modest means and, compared to the patients on DeBakey's service, modest problems.

So, on Saturday mornings around 6:30 a.m., Bud would leave Rachel and their cozy cottage in the Montrose area and travel the few miles to Crawford's spacious home in River Oaks. They'd go out for a big breakfast and strong coffee somewhere, and then start "doing cases," as Bud puts it. Often, the only other doctor in attendance would be a family practitioner; itinerant surgery, as it was called then, is now illegal. But here was how Bud learned to be a surgeon, assisting Crawford in taking out gallbladders and repairing small-bowel blockages, whatever was needed. Crawford never raised his voice; he was exacting but patient. There was no other place on earth Bud would rather have been.

Even so, he had already decided to specialize in heart surgery. The death toll from heart disease was skyrocketing in 1963: every day another patient at Methodist died because the doctors had so little to offer. There was one patient in particular whose terrified, pleading expression would stay with Bud for the rest of his life. He had worked up a medical history for one of DeBakey's growing list of international patients, a seventeen-year-old Italian boy who was only a few years younger than Bud himself. Med students who did the workup also got to scrub in on the patient's surgery. Bud was there for what he expected to be a routine replacement of a damaged aortic valve. The kid was thin from his illness but handsome, with dark eyes and thick black hair; optimistic about the surgery, he was eager to go back home. His mother was with him.

The surgery went fine—Bud held and retracted, nothing glamorous, but still exciting for a student. That night, though, the boy's heart stopped—this sometimes happened, inexplicably, with aortic valve disease. The only way to save the boy was to use a procedure that had first been tried just two years back, in 1961—to reopen the chest and manually massage the heart to restart it.

A resident cut the boy open again, then turned to the strongest person in the room: Bud. He showed Bud how to reach into the boy's chest and squeeze his heart, mimicking the pumping action of a healthy organ. Around that time, the sedated boy woke up and locked eyes with Bud. The nurses sedated him again, but the boy kept his gaze on Bud and tried to reach for him, to hold on. Minutes passed. Bud's hands cramped, and then the pain began radiating up his arm. He kept going.

DeBakey strode in, took one look at the scene, and ordered Bud to stop. Experience told him that too much time had passed, and that they were not going to be able to restart the boy's heart. But Bud kept squeezing and releasing, until finally a resident had to shove him aside. As soon as Bud let go, the boy slipped away. He could hear the mother sobbing in the waiting room when DeBakey went out to give her the news.

As it turned out, that episode would change everything for Bud. If the simple pumping action of his hand could keep someone alive, he figured, there should be some kind of machine that could do it longer and better. It would have to be something a tech could pull off the shelf and a surgeon could implant, a machine that would run almost perpetually inside a human chest. An artificial heart.

A TOUR OF HELL

"It's too painful and it's really not that important," Bud says about his military service. Still, his one-year tour in Vietnam does come up every once in a while. He likes going to author readings, and if the author is a veteran, Bud is likely to add his own commentary at some length, during the Q&A session for which he has often arrived late. He is a fan of Viet Thanh Nguyen's "The Sympathizer," for instance, but took umbrage at Nguyen's meditation on war, "Nothing Ever Dies." "That guy was never in combat," he snorted, providing a capsule review.

Bud's personal philosophy of war is that young men are sent to fight because old generals need something to do. On this subject he likes to quote the cynical old saw from a probably mythical general who told his troops: "Boys, this is a bad war, but it's the only one we've got."

Exhibit A is a DVD entitled *Bud Frazier's Holiday in Vietnam*, made for a biographical film about his life that was never produced. Frazier tends to watch it leaning way back in his office chair, with his hands on his belly, the look on his face not quite readable—wonder? pride?—as he watches a version of himself from more than fifty years ago, sporting a buzz cut and deep dimples when he grins. Then as now, he has a sly look in his eyes that suggests more than a passing acquaintance with and deep affection for absurdity.

The silent, one-hour video is a collection of clips that span the time from November 1968 until the end of 1969, when Bud's tour was up. Judging from the content, he seems to have spent the year ministering to villagers, especially apprehensive children, and learning karate from the Korean soldiers his unit was supposed to be training. In the video, he works for his black belt by practicing complex spins and high kicks that land perilously close to the chin of his instructor. There Bud is, tall, tanned, and impossibly buff—his grown daughter, Allison, would later tease that he was never that thin. There are shots of boat rides up and down a stunning coastline lined with white sand beaches and palm trees, the jungle-covered mountains in the distance. In other scenes, Bud places his stethoscope on the chests of wary children while a gaggle of villagers wearing paddy hats surround him, pushing forward to be next in line. Bud was twenty-eight when he was drafted—just in the middle of his residency in general surgery. Still, in those moments, the lanky, easygoing West Texan disappears. His body grows tight and coiled, as if he is dispatching all his concentration to the fingertips holding his stethoscope in place. The surgeon he will become is plainly visible, his confidence and concentration amid the chaos almost palpable.

Bud was drafted as part of the Berry Plan, a federal program that was supposed to address the shortage of doctors in the military by offering plum assignments. The government asked medical draftees to list their top three preferred placements. Bud was no dummy; he requested surgery jobs in Hawaii, San Francisco, or Germany. The officer in charge started laughing when Bud told him he hadn't requested Vietnam.

Still, Bud figured he had a way out. One of his closest friends from medical school was from the Texas-Mexico border near Del

Rio, the son of a wealthy radio station owner who ran one of the cuckoo, buy-our-autographed-pictures-of-Jesus channels that proliferated back then. He'd also grown up accustomed to the kind of hazy legality that was part of life on the border, so he convinced Bud he could bribe his way out of Vietnam. The guy knew a guy—an officer in Washington, DC, they could talk to. When they got their meeting, they headed for the nation's capital. In a result that could only shock a pair of twentysomethings, that officer also started laughing when they made their offer.

Bud's next sidestep was to follow the advice of a returned veteran who was running the Baylor charity hospital at the time: Bud should apply to become a flight surgeon, because he would make an extra $100 a month and would get training in aerospace medicine. This sounded like a great idea, so that's what Bud did.

He finished training school in the fall and headed for Saigon, armed with a copy of Marcus Aurelius' *Meditations*, a paean to stoicism his aunt had given Bud just before he left home. He would need it.

His base camp was near Na Trang in the Central Highlands, the scene, along with the Mekong Delta, of some of the worst fighting in the war. Bud's unit consisted of about three hundred men, mostly young—eighteen was the average age—mostly poor, and mostly of color, a microcosm of the US soldiers who fought in the war. Because Bud was all of twenty-eight, the boys called him Dad. He was one of two with a college education. The other was a fresh-faced graduate of UCLA who wanted to be a journalist, and thought a tour in Vietnam would be a great training ground.

There was a lot of downtime. Bud took in the stories of his fellow soldiers, and the uneasy relationship between the Korean and the Vietnamese troops. He tamed a pet lemur with orange slices, and learned to speak Vietnamese with a West Texas accent. He made beds for some kids in an orphanage, who continued to sleep on the floor. When Bud's son Todd was born six months into his tour, he showed the pictures around and got plenty of props. "They say it's very good fortune to have your first child as a boy," he told Rachel in one of the tape-recorded letters they sent to each other. In the early days, Bud's voice is soft and supple with humor and wonder, his descriptions sometimes set to the strings of Vietnamese café music or the sound of incoming helicopters.

That was the hint that the romance of war was fleeting. Bud's job, among others, was to identify the men killed in his unit; the US Army didn't want families missing death benefits because their loved ones were wrongly and indefinitely classified as MIAs. Soon enough, Bud was jumping on and off helicopters, riding to battle scenes, and helping to pull the dead and wounded off the field.

A helicopter in the middle of a battle is no place anyone wants to be. The wounded boys screamed to the *thwamp thwamp thwamp* of the rotor blades. The gunner returned fire from his assault rifle so close to the ground that the pings of enemy bullets blew tiny circles of light into the helicopter's metal sides. The chopper pitched and bucked as the pilot tried to avoid being shot down, and the sharp, metallic smell of blood was everywhere.

In that chaos, Bud's job was to stitch up the soldiers and start IVs as fast as he could. They were his friends: he'd dodged mortar rounds at camp with them, played cards and shared beers with them, heard about their mothers and fathers, wives and girlfriends, sons and daughters. Soon enough, he found himself wondering over morning coffee who wouldn't come back at the end of the day.

Or who he would find with an arm or a leg blown off, or a hole in the head where an eye or an ear should have been. Blood spurted everywhere in the helicopters, cracked bones pushed through the skin—by the time Bud got back to base, he would be covered with crimson spatters and lost bits of muscle and flesh. Every mission was a mystery: Bud never knew what kind of damage he would find; he just jumped out of the chopper and grabbed whoever or whatever he could while the bullets flew. Sometimes it was too late—Bud would find the boy from New York or Indiana dead on a mountainside. All he could do was zip the soldier into a black body bag for his last ride home.

The dense, triple-canopy mountains had few good roads, and the North Vietnamese soldiers knew their way around much better than the GIs. Days were okay, but at night, no one left the compound because the Vietcong were always waiting just outside the perimeter. Sometimes Bud suspected his unit was dispatched just to flush out the enemy. The helicopters' noisy clumsiness made them easy targets.

The American government kept secret its knowledge that the war was unwinnable as early as 1965, but it didn't take Bud long to come to the same conclusion during his tour. The corruption required to fight the war was one indication—it seemed the South Vietnamese always required a payoff for anything Bud needed. He could see that the Vietnamese people didn't really want the Americans there, and the more he treated the men in his unit for venereal diseases, the more he came to understand why. It reminded him of his days playing football for a neighboring West Texas high school team; all the local boys hated him for his arrogance, for taking their girls, for acting like a conqueror when he wasn't any such thing.

Bud to this day describes his commander "as big a redneck as you will ever see." It wasn't surprising that he took an instant dislike to his college-boy doctor, either—he was sure Bud wasn't owning up to being a Jew. Bud had been a good soldier to DeBakey back in Houston; DeBakey had been demanding, and maybe a little nuts, but he had never asked his troops to do anything stupid. Now Bud was being asked to report soldiers for smoking dope—"Of course they were," Bud would say—and he refused. Soon after that, the commanding officer began sending him on ever more dangerous missions. Twice the VC shot out the engine of his helicopter, and the pilot had to land without power.

On another sweltering, sunny day, Bud was driving an ambulance back from a hospital near Cam Ranh Bay. Up ahead he spotted what looked like bodies on the dusty road, some moving, some not. As he drew closer, Bud realized they'd hit a land mine. The small group had been riding one of those oversized tricycles common in Vietnam, half a dozen or so men, women, and children hanging on to the handlebars and crammed into baskets. Now they were blown to bits.

Bud jumped out and started some IVs he had in the truck—people were bleeding and screaming all around him. In his haste, he left his .45 on the driver's seat of the ambulance, and someone snatched it. Bud's commander used the incident to start a court-martial, which, luckily, went nowhere. Around that time, his closest friend, the would-be journalist from California, was killed in the fighting. He was shot through the neck while riding home on the helicopter. In Bud's tape-recorded account of his loss to Rachel, his voice is stilted and flat, like a robot's. By then, he also had a notebook full of poems with titles like "The Body Bag" and "An American Boy," a paean to a dead comrade.

It was a very long tour.

Bud returned to Rachel, finally met six-month-old Todd, and took his place back in DeBakey's general surgery residency. He didn't tell anyone what he was feeling, which was nothing. When Rachel asked him about Vietnam, all Bud would say was that he had seen so many lives wasted that he wanted to dedicate the rest of his to saving as many people as he could.

Bud's father had gone to fight in World War II when Bud was three and had come back a stranger, never quite able to reconnect, never able to talk about what he'd seen. Now Bud understood. If he had always been solitary, now he was more so. When he wasn't working, he spent his free time at a folk bar, Anderson Fair, listening to music, adrift. He did not always make it home. Rachel whispered to friends that the husband who had gone off to war was not the same man who had come back.

Bud had always been a voracious reader, but now he carried dog-eared, well-thumbed paperbacks—something classic or obscure, never a bestseller—in his lab coat pocket like a shield. He was often reading, or appearing to read, while shuffling through the hospital corridors in a way that kept others away. In staff meetings or during grand rounds, he sat in the back, sometimes with a book open, never quite present. And then he would rejoin the world with an incisive comment or offer an esoteric fact before going back to his book, rolling back into himself like some raggedy magic carpet.

"Be like a rocky promontory against which the restless surf continually pounds; it stands fast while the churning sea is lulled to sleep at its feet," begins a passage from Marcus Aurelius that best describes Bud at that time. "I hear you say, 'How unlucky that this should happen to me!' Not at all! Say instead, 'How lucky that I am not broken by what has happened and am not afraid of what is about to happen. The same blow might have struck anyone, but not many would have absorbed it without capitulation or complaint.'"

—⁓—

To be under DeBakey's thumb was all-consuming—you just did what you were told and kept your head down. If you were assigned to the intensive care unit, you didn't leave the hospital for three months. If your child was born during that time, too bad. If it was Christmas Eve, sorry: you celebrated alone, with fried pies and Fritos or whatever else you could scrounge from the cafeteria. As one doctor would later tell author Tommy Thompson in his chronicle of the Cooley-DeBakey feud *Hearts*, "I got a vitamin deficiency and my tongue turned fire red. I figured that what I went through was the supreme test of human endurance."

Bud didn't see it that way. The ICU was dark and quiet, except for the beeping of monitors and the occasional emergency, which he handled with ease. It was the perfect place for someone who did not want to think about where he had been or what he had seen. After all, he wasn't under fire, and he wasn't trying to stitch up a screaming teenager in a lurching, bucking helicopter. Still, when a pregnant Rachel brought Todd to visit during the off-hours, Bud was usually too tired to take much note; he could barely stay awake long enough to bounce his son on his knee.

The end of his term in the ICU didn't offer much relief. The brutal Baylor call schedule still required thirty-six hours on duty and twelve hours off, which wasn't much time to recover, even for a strong, stubborn thirty-year-old man. If DeBakey believed medical training should mimic the battlefield, Bud couldn't argue: keeping himself in a world of trauma was, if not the safest place, then at least the most familiar. There was always someone begging to be saved.

But despite his own fog of war, Bud was still determined to be a heart surgeon, and he'd figured out that DeBakey wasn't giving interns much action in his operating room. He had far too many good surgeons on his staff to let an amateur practice on his patients, even if they had been trained by Michael DeBakey, at Michael DeBakey's medical school, and even if their combat experience trumped his. Bud found himself drawn to the neighboring Texas Heart Institute, which after only eight or so years in business was doing more heart surgery than any other place in the world. That was because it was run by Denton Cooley, who by the late 1960s was gaining on De-Bakey for the title of world's most famous heart surgeon.

In the highly competitive if still tiny world of heart surgery, Cooley was believed to have no equal. Watching him operate was like watching a master magician: even if you knew how a trick was done, you couldn't possibly duplicate it. But Cooley had also gone to UT and distinguished himself as an athlete, like Bud. He was known to be a risk taker, someone who would try anything to save a patient, like Bud. As an added plus, Cooley had never, in Bud's recollection, called anyone on his service a moron.

Bud figured that he could do his residency in cardiac surgery at Texas Heart and then go back to work for DeBakey. He was still committed to creating an artificial heart, and he knew Cooley didn't have much interest in research.

It was a reasonable plan. There was just no way in hell it was going to work out, because Cooley and DeBakey were at war.

THE WAR AT HOME

If you were going to invent someone who was, in almost every way, the polar opposite of Michael DeBakey, it would be Denton Cooley. DeBakey was homely, cerebral, and hotheaded under pressure, which was virtually all of the time. He was a child of immigrants, with all the pressures that entailed. He wore lifts in his white English surgical boots. He was impatient and high-handed when he wasn't charming the likes of Mary Lasker or Lyndon Baines Johnson.

Cooley, on the other hand, was from a prominent Houston family, best buddies with the sons and daughters of business and oil barons, the movers and shakers who made the city go. Tall and thin, with an athlete's easy grace, he had eyes the pale blue of robin's eggs and a toothy, rakish grin. Cooley was so handsome that even the starchiest operating room nurses could become giggling schoolgirls in his presence. He could make the wives of patients momentarily forget their husbands' dire circumstances. His nickname was "Dr. Wonderful." In the operating room, he did not throw instruments or tantrums; he was fast, dexterous, and inventive; he loved the unexpected disaster, which is all too common in heart surgery. He seemed to be, at least to the residents and interns on his service, always in control.

And Cooley had a real life outside of the hospital. DeBakey made it to his oldest son's wedding in Peru only after his staff surreptitiously scheduled some lectures there. Cooley put in endless hours at the hospital, but photographs of his wife and five blond daughters decorated his office, and he took time off with the family at his ranch an hour or so from Houston. They called it Cool Acres.

The goals of DeBakey and Cooley were different too. DeBakey was a force of nature, a determined, relentless change agent. Cooley wanted to be the best surgeon who ever lived, period. During the early 1960s, when peace still reigned between them (more or less), the two Houston doctors were so famous that a popular television show called *Ben Casey* was based on their lives, and made their differences abundantly clear: Ben Casey was the darkly handsome and hip young surgeon, while his mentor, the peculiar and ethnic Dr. Zorba, was played by a much older, much shorter, much balder actor whose remaining hair had the texture of a beat-up Brillo pad. As time went on, the main difference between real life and television was that Zorba and Casey got along.

But for all his superficial ease and all his confounding gifts, Cooley was a complex man every bit as determined and competitive as his nemesis. In fact, he was expert at holding a grudge. Charmingly.

Cooley's autobiography, *100,000 Hearts*, offers an insight into his thinking. The title comes from the number of hearts Cooley operated on in his long career. Who's counting? you might ask. He was. Despite a rich and successful career, Cooley was obsessive about keeping score.

That predilection had to have come from his 1920s Texas childhood. Cooley's grandfather had made a fortune in real estate. Both his son Ralph and the East Texas beauty he married, Mary Fraley, were curious, cultured people—Mary especially loved to play the piano for company almost as much as she doted on her sons, Ralph Jr. and Denton, who was sixteen months younger than his brother. Ralph senior's dental practice grew quickly because of the family's prominence; he had intended to become a doctor, but an episode of hazing at the University of Texas put an end to his plans. For Denton, this may have been a good thing: when the senior Cooley wasn't treating some of Houston's most illustrious citizens, he retreated to his workshop, where he busied himself inventing dental instruments. Often he recruited Denton to help, and early on the boy showed a talent for fashioning tools and casting gold teeth.

Mostly, though, Cooley's youth was unfettered in the way that so many Texans valued, and still value, above all else. He and his brother roamed the city at will. They rode their bikes across town to their grandparents' turreted Victorian mansion in the Houston Heights, pedaling north from their modest brick bungalow in Montrose, dodging the streetcar on wide, magnolia-shaded Heights Boulevard. The brothers swam and fished in the bayous around town, and hunted birds and squirrels with their own shotguns. They plundered the orchard of one local oilman—"Our fig raids may have taught us a questionable lesson: stolen fruit is sweeter than store-bought," Cooley later wrote—and borrowed golf clubs from neighborhood garages, playing for free on public golf courses. "Although the green fee was only fifty cents," Cooley noted, "we were disinclined to pay it."

They became experts at siphoning gas too—like most Texans of his time, Cooley got his driver's license at thirteen, and saved money to buy his own Model T a few years later by delivering newspapers. (His dog Jack rode on the running board.) Cooley seemed to know instinctively how to keep the car running smoothly, his strong hands and long, deft fingers tightening the hoses and replacing belts with the confidence of an experienced mechanic. When Cooley couldn't find a ready-made part, he made one himself.

Still, his life wasn't trouble-free. Ralph Cooley Sr. was a drinker, and when he'd had too much he showed off a nasty temper. He beat his wife and tore into his sons. When the Cooley boys went off to college, their parents divorced, an uncommon practice in the 1930s. Cooley would note in his autobiography that in the aftermath neither parent "ever regained their rightful social standing." Ralph's professional life and health deteriorated as he drank more; Mary married unsuccessfully two more times, and finally changed her name back to Cooley.

The years of family strife left Denton with scars that were invisible but significant. He'd learned to keep his innermost thoughts and dreams to himself, the hallmarks of a man who decided early on that trust was negotiable and of dubious benefit. And that he was, mostly, on his own.

Cooley's abundant gifts easily obscured whatever inner demons he harbored. While his brother became a life-of-the-party type at the University of Texas and later descended into alcoholism, Cooley slipped effortlessly into the role of golden boy: he played varsity basketball and, as a fraternity brother, extended his network of wealthy and accomplished friends, who would one day become the state's lawyers, engineers, oilmen, and politicians as well as his patients. Cooley managed to be both a team player and a star on and off the court, a dashing ladies' man who was revered by his fraternity brothers and who graduated with honors, seemingly without breaking a sweat. ("The lowest grades I made during my four years at UT were two B's," he was still noting, seventy or so years after he graduated.)

Cooley's maternal grandfather had been a doctor, and there were his father's frustrated medical ambitions to contend with. Cooley headed for medical school at the University of Texas Medical Branch in Galveston, but in 1942 transferred to Johns Hopkins in Baltimore, then considered the best and most enlightened medical school in the United States. Once there, he became a favorite of the chief of surgery, Alfred Blalock, one of the preeminent surgeons in the country. Among other things, he admired Cooley's skill at ping-pong.

Intentionally or not, the young Dr. Cooley had perfected a veneer of cool. But, in fact, he was already determined to turn himself into a great surgeon. He took string to his room at night and practiced tying knots faster and faster, first with two hands, then with one. He worked with a scalpel and pieces of meat to find just the right way to hold his fingers in surgery to make the best cut. The more Cooley studied, the more he was drawn to the heart. A handful of doctors were just beginning to unravel its mysteries, and he felt a call to work in a field where the ground had barely been turned.

In the 1940s, Cooley soon came up against the same problem that flummoxed DeBakey and his colleagues: you could work around the heart, but you couldn't get inside it. No one had any idea how to stop the heart and repair it without killing the patient. A defective valve or a weakness in the muscle was usually a death sentence.

At the time, Blalock had a very unusual partnership with a gifted black man named Vivien Thomas. Blalock had met Thomas in 1929 as a medical student at the Vanderbilt University hospital, when Thomas was working as a carpenter. Thomas had hoped to go to college and medical school himself, but the failure of a Nashville bank during the Great Depression wiped out his savings—and because he was black, his options were further limited. White schools had yet to become interested in turning out black doctors, and there were only two black colleges in the United States that offered medical training.

Blalock invited Thomas to become his "surgical technician," a misnomer for the word "partner." Thomas' extraordinary gifts at surgery became quickly apparent, and it wasn't long before he was running Blalock's research lab, trying out new techniques on dogs. The times being what they were, Thomas continued to be classified as a janitor on the payroll.

Over the next few years, the two men did groundbreaking work on the causes of shock, saving countless lives on the battlefields of World War II by proving Blalock's theory that loss of fluid in the blood vessels, not toxins in the blood, caused the body to go into shock. (Hence the IVs Bud would start on the battlefields of Vietnam decades later.)

But Blalock and Thomas were mostly concerned with breaking the last medical taboo: cutting into the heart itself. Soon they began causing heart defects in dogs so they could learn how to repair them.

In 1941, they had help from a brilliant Hopkins pediatric cardiologist by the name of Helen Taussig, who was then developing a theory of her own about a condition known as "blue baby syndrome," a birth defect in which newborns turned blue because of a lack of oxygen and died within minutes. Taussig theorized that the problem was caused either by a partial blockage in the pulmonary artery and valve (a superhighway that carries freshly oxygenated blood from the right ventricle to the lungs) or by a hole that caused leakage between the ventricles of an infant's heart—or maybe by some combination of both. Taussig thought the condition, commonly known as Tetralogy of Fallot, could be corrected surgically. She took her ideas to the august surgeon Robert Gross, who, not surprisingly—Taussig was a girl, after all—ignored her. So Taussig turned to Blalock and Thomas, who were not so dismissive. Blalock, in fact, said he had been thinking exactly along those lines.

In 1944, Blalock and Thomas tried the surgery on a dying baby, with Blalock holding the knife and Thomas telling him where to cut. They worked in a chilly operating room lit by two large windows and heated by cast-iron radiators. They had asked for volunteers, and one intern eagerly stepped up: twenty-four-year-old Denton Cooley. The surgery, in which they created an artificial passageway that joined the two major arteries that allow blood to flow from the heart into the lungs, took ninety minutes. Blalock removed a final clamp, and it was as if he had repaired a leak in a garden hose: as the heart began pumping normally, the blood began flowing normally, and the grayish-blue infant on the operating table turned a rosy pink.

The operation wasn't a complete success—the baby died soon after of further complications. But for Denton Cooley, it was a turning point: he had seen for himself the drama, the risk, and the profound potential of a brand-new field, and he wanted in.

—∿∿—

Cooley reported for his first day of work as Baylor College of Medicine's first chief of cardiovascular surgery on June 1, 1951. Even for a native Houstonian like him, the atmosphere could not have been pleasant. Jefferson Davis Hospital was an Art Deco monolith adjacent to Houston's Buffalo Bayou—it looked a lot like a twelve-story Depression-era state capitol—and inside, the temperatures and the humidity would have been even higher, given the lack of air-conditioning. The halls were crowded with patients on stretchers and slumped in wheelchairs; they were mostly black, virtually all of them poor. At the time, Jeff Davis was Houston's only charity hospital, and like charity hospitals everywhere at the time, it exemplified certain antebellum and pre-Medicaid attitudes about the less fortunate. Sometimes there were as many rats and roaches scurrying in the hallways as nurses.

DeBakey, however, believed medical care was a right, not a privilege. Three years into his efforts to rebuild Baylor, he had already commandeered Jeff Davis as one of the medical school's first teaching hospitals. Its cadavers went to the anatomy studies, while the surviving members of Houston's indigent population were suddenly graced with a profound uptick in their medical care—in exchange for serving as guinea pigs for Baylor interns. Accustomed to the hell of New Orleans' Charity Hospital and battlefield hospital tents, De-Bakey was oblivious to the misery around him, except as it applied to his ability to relieve it. He flew through the hospital halls, his white-coated entourage flapping like hapless gulls behind him.

On Cooley's first day, DeBakey had gathered this small group around the bedside of a patient named Mitchell, whose first name has been lost. He was forty-six, but not a young forty-six, crippled as he was by an aneurysm of the aortic arch—in layman's terms, a dangerous weakening of the arterial wall where it curves just above the heart. If the artery burst, the patient would die within minutes. DeBakey's medical team had already tried the treatment of choice, wrapping the artery in cellophane to support the weakened wall, but the technique wasn't helping. Weak, winded, and unable to move, Mr. Mitchell seemed to have run out of options.

DeBakey greeted the man with a warmth he seldom showed his underlings. Then he turned to the patient's chart, flipped through it, checked Mr. Mitchell's vitals, and stopped to ponder, seemingly in the grip of a novel idea. Abruptly DeBakey fixed his owl eyes on the newest member of his team and asked what he would do for the poor man.

Cooley answered without hesitation: the patient needed surgery to cut out the aneurysm. Everyone had a good chuckle over that, because no one had *ever* removed an aneurysm. It wasn't done. You used the cellophane wrap and hoped for the best. Everyone knew that.

Except, apparently, Denton Cooley, who at thirty-one was fresh from training in what were quite possibly the best hospitals in the world. After graduating in 1945 from Hopkins, he fulfilled his military service by running a small hospital in Linz, Austria, for three years, and then eagerly returned to Baltimore, where he was enshrined as chief resident on the Hopkins cardiac service until he finished his training in 1950.

By that time, the most advanced surgeons knew from experience on the battlefield that the heart might be more receptive to repair than was previously known. One surgeon removed bits of shrapnel embedded in a wounded soldier's heart, and the patient made a complete recovery. Other doctors had been able to reach and repair minor damage to the mitral valve, one of the most important regulators of blood flow into the left ventricle. Cooley, like the handful of others in his field, could sense that heart surgery was coming into its own.

DeBakey had heard of Cooley's skills and had recruited him for Baylor; Cooley went because oilman Hugh Roy Cullen had just donated $22 million to the school, a good indication that big things were going to happen. DeBakey agreed to hold Cooley's job for a year while he studied at London's illustrious Brompton Hospital with Russell Brock, one of the most accomplished heart surgeons of the time. Everything seemed to be falling into place: Cooley had married Louise Thomas, a pert, pretty surgical nurse and the daughter of a prominent Maryland physician, and they already had a little girl named Mary.

Now, however, Michael DeBakey was treating him like a rube. Worse, DeBakey had done it before. Back in 1945, Cooley had hoped to fulfill his military requirement by working at Walter Reed Army Hospital, in Washington, DC. He hand-carried Blalock's recommendation letter to the surgeon general's office, where he encountered a pretentious officer who took the letter and, Cooley always believed, torpedoed his chances. But he wasn't going to let DeBakey thwart him again. Maybe putting up with his father's abuse gave Cooley an edge over more easily intimidated doctors.

The patient needed an aneurysmectomy, Cooley now argued,

persisting. You cut out the weakened portion of the arterial wall and then sew the aorta back together. Cooley had done two such procedures at Hopkins. "He sure doesn't have a chance lying here in bed," Cooley added, grimly eyeing the patient.

DeBakey turned on his heel and swept out of the room as if he had never asked a question at all, much less heard the answer. But later that day he sent Cooley a message: he should schedule the aneurysmectomy for nine-thirty the next morning. That night, Cooley raced across town to the VA hospital to grab some surgical tools unavailable at Jeff Davis—a chisel and special mallet. The next morning, he was just finishing when DeBakey burst into the OR, gowned and gloved, as if he had been called to assist in an emergency.

There wasn't one. Mr. Mitchell recovered and went home. DeBakey published a paper on the procedure, and got himself lauded, not for the first time, as an intrepid and inventive surgeon. He rewarded his new surgical head by omitting Cooley's name from the paper—stingy, but DeBakey's right as chief—and then sent Cooley seven hundred cases to review. Cooley stashed the files in a drawer and, like DeBakey, forgot about them.

—⁓—

For a while, Cooley appeared to adopt a "forgive and remember" attitude toward DeBakey. Houston was already building a reputation as the most innovative center of heart surgery in the world, thanks to the two men. Papers by Cooley and DeBakey—written separately and together—were coveted by medical journals. They toured— separately and together—Europe, Asia, and South America, lecturing at medical schools and showing off their latest techniques. Those exhibitions also served as excellent marketing tools for drawing still more patients to Houston, accompanied as the visits were by breathless press accounts.

Fortunately, the two surgeons didn't do exactly the same thing. DeBakey was a vascular surgeon—he worked on the arteries and veins around the heart—while also serving as a masterful lobbyist for public health. Cooley was completely focused and utterly fearless in his approach to the terra incognita of the heart. When one reporter suggested he might be taking too many risks, Cooley was ready with a response: "I'm often obliged to experiment inside the heart of a patient whose problem hasn't yet been worked out in a dog."

Central to the progress of heart surgery, Cooley believed, was a machine that could keep the blood oxygenated and circulating through the body long enough for a surgeon to operate on the heart—something that worked on the heart's circulatory system like a bypass on a highway. Cooley was already known for his velocity in the operating room—his autobiography is replete with record-breaking speeds for operations—but some complex repairs were still beyond his nearly superhuman skills.

Heart surgery in its beginnings and for subsequent decades would continue to be brutal, coarse, and rudimentary. There was nothing like an MRI or even effective cardiac catheterization to help a surgeon identify the problem. Once he began to cut, he was essentially flying blind. Just getting to the heart was something of an ordeal, for doctor and patient—a procedure known as a full median sternotomy. The surgeon made an incision into the sternum, and then put his index finger in the sternal notch, the space between the neck and collarbones. Then he took what's called a sternal saw and cut through the sternum, separating the breastbone in two and steadying it with a retractor. Sometimes, in the process, a surgeon would break a rib with the retractor, and sometimes he would accidentally cut into the pericardium, the membrane covering the heart, or even, unfortunately, the heart itself. Even today, with so much technology, surgeons can never be sure what they will find. "The heart will al-ways surprise you," is something of a cliché for a reason.

Nowadays, the heart-lung machine is an elaborate and exacting device that keeps both organs functioning while the heart goes off line for surgery. But in the earliest days cardiac surgeons had nothing like that. They had to imagine what a device like that would look like, and how it would function. Cooley wanted something better than the machine John Gibbon had begun to develop with the help of IBM in the 1930s. Other doctors were making improvements to the original device, and Cooley thought it would be a great idea to bring such a machine to Baylor. He went to DeBakey with the pros-pect. The response: no thanks. DeBakey and his team were already working on their version of the heart-lung machine. He did not ask Cooley to help out.

So Cooley struck out on his own. He traveled to Minnesota to meet with Walt Lillehei and Richard DeWall, who in 1955 were also working on a heart-lung machine. In this device, blood from the patient flowed through tubes into a container where it was exposed to bubbles of oxygen, then "defoamed"—air bubbles were fatal—and returned through a helix-shaped coil to the patient's body. The results were promising. (By that point, Lillehei was also well into a hard-partying phase. He took Cooley to a roadhouse for a very long night, and then prepared for surgery the next morning by having a nurse pop an amyl nitrate capsule under his nose. Lillehei's hell-bent-for-leather leanings made him an early role model for the first heart surgeons as much as Chuck Yeager was for *The Right Stuff* test pilots. Yeager, however, was never prosecuted for failing to pay his taxes.)

Cooley imported the machine to Houston, just in time to re-spond to a desperate plea from a colleague who had a patient with a hole in the wall, or septum, between the left and right ventricles. His only chance to live was open-heart surgery, but even Cooley wouldn't be able to perform this kind of operation without some kind of mechanical help.

The year was 1957, and the number of open-heart surgeries that had been performed in the United States up to that time amounted to a meager fifty. Cooley doesn't write about how long it took him to decide to operate, but anyone who knew him would guess somewhere in the neighborhood of two seconds. He connected the patient to the pump and then sewed up several tears he found in the septum ("I managed to do the entire procedure in only twenty-five minutes of cardiopulmonary bypass time, which was quite a feat in such a complicated case"). The patient lived for six more weeks; then, as happened often in the early days of heart surgery, he died of an infection.

Still, Cooley saw the operation as an enormous success. "We were in the open-heart business," he would write. News spread quickly among other cardiologists and surgeons, and Cooley's office was flooded with referrals. After all, a slight chance of survival was better than none.

But Cooley knew he could improve on the original, and decided to build his own machine. This being Houston, he got an oil broker pal on the phone and explained he wanted to build a heart-lung machine and sure could use some help. He might as well have been asking for a home improvement loan: Cooley's friend promptly sent over a check for $5,000. Then Cooley, with the help of three associates, headed to a local hardware store, bought the parts he needed, and had them all fabricated into a heart-lung contraption at a place called Commercial Kitchens, where, of course, Cooley was a friend of the owner. What he designed was a smaller version of Lillehei's machine, one that could be easily sterilized and that more effectively removed air bubbles from the blood. It was nicknamed the "Cooley Coffeepot" because it looked like a percolator. Within four months,

Cooley had used his device successfully thirty-nine times. By the end of that year, he had performed more open-heart surgeries than anyone else on the planet.

DeBakey had kept close tabs on Cooley's progress—his own heart-lung machine hadn't gotten very far. He scheduled an operation on a child with a heart defect, intending to use Cooley's machine and Cooley's team—but not Cooley. That plan did not go over well. Cooley complained that DeBakey had no right to schedule an operation using his device and his people without his permission. DeBakey was unmoved: Cooley, he claimed, had created the machine while on the Baylor faculty. Cooley countered that he had raised the money privately. Uncharacteristically, DeBakey backed down and allowed Cooley to do the surgery, which, given the differences in their age and technology know-how, was probably a smart idea.

The operation was successful, and once again patients clamored for Cooley's touch. By the beginning of 1959, he had performed six hundred successful operations using the heart-lung bypass machine. With more refinements, Cooley began performing ever more complex surgeries that had never been done before—treating calcified aortic valves and correcting previously fatal congenital defects, along with rare aneurysms and pulmonary embolisms (blood clots in the lungs). Cooley and his heart-lung machine were in such demand that he could sometimes be seen carting it from one hospital in the Texas Medical Center to another in the family station wagon with the help of his wife, Louise.

To Cooley, the invention and popularization of the heart-lung bypass marked the true beginnings of heart surgery: "The first time in history that this mysterious muscular organ, the source of life's pulse, could be arrested, cut open, repaired, closed and restarted," as he put it.

But it also marked another step in the deterioration of the relationship between the powerful Baylor chief and his equally ambitious protégé. Relations had grown so testy that everyone from scrub nurses to international socialites began to feel as though they had to choose sides. Mary Lasker wrote of one particular evening when Cooley and DeBakey made a joint appearance: "Denton Cooley, another surgeon from Houston, was there, who was very attractive but didn't have the big statesmanlike quality that DeBakey has. . . . Cooley is a fantastically skilled surgeon that Princess Lilian [of Belgium] also took a great fancy to, but he is strictly parochial Texas as far as politics or health insurance goes."

Parochial or no, the census at DeBakey's most prized Baylor affiliated hospital, Methodist, was exploding. Its popularity was certainly due to DeBakey's reputation, but now also to Cooley's. A silent battle for hospital beds and operating rooms between Baylor's biggest stars naturally followed. Tired of DeBakey's bigfooting and always eager for more room for more patients, Cooley quietly moved most of his operations out of DeBakey's reach without abandoning the Texas Medical Center. His first perch was Texas Children's Hospital— Cooley did perform surgery on children and infants, after all—and then, in 1960, he moved to St. Luke's Episcopal Hospital nearby.

—◣◢—

Cooley began building a world in his image. He populated his formal office at St. Luke's with stunning nurses and secretaries, leggy and mostly blond, who called his patients "sweetheart" and "darlin." They wore short skirts and sometimes took notes using ballpoint pens topped with artificial daisies. The residents who assisted were also uniformly attractive—virile Texas good ole boys—as if Cooley were assembling his team by way of central casting.

When he wasn't operating, Cooley spent most of his time in a small, cluttered, windowless office near Operating Room 1. Every day, he made quick work of the same disciplined lunch—a cup of yogurt or soup and half a sandwich—and thought about what he wanted.

Cooley felt the pressure: People were dying because advances in treating and curing heart disease weren't coming fast enough. And the number of sufferers was going up, particularly for middle-aged white men. For those whose hearts he could not repair, he had nothing. There were only two answers: someone had to come up with a way to transplant a heart from one person to another, or someone had to come up with a mechanical replacement for the heart.

A mechanical heart, Cooley thought, just wasn't feasible. He'd heard scuttlebutt from Methodist that DeBakey believed that if a damaged heart was just given a rest—helped along with a mechanical pump—it would eventually cure itself, a premise Cooley found absurd. Other heart surgeons, however, were not so sure. The brilliant surgeon Adrian Kantrowitz, who had devised his own heart-lung machine, had also worked with a colleague at Maimonides Hospital in Brooklyn to transfer some muscle from a dog's diaphragm into its damaged heart. That healthy muscle was able to take over 25 percent of the heart's pumping action, thanks to an electric booster from the natural pulsations, transferred via radio signal. (The dog, named Ruff, was a mutt who was later named Research Dog of the Year by the New York Academy of Sciences for his contribution to medical progress.)

Cooley was far more interested in the second option, transplantation. Yes, there were problems of tissue rejection, but those, he believed, were no big deal. He was more frustrated by psychological barriers. Transplants raised all kinds of questions with—to him—varying degrees of looniness among the public: Could a person still get into heaven with the heart of another? Would a man become more feminine if he received the heart of a woman? And so on. It infuriated the preternaturally pragmatic Cooley that so many people still believed the heart was the center of the soul, and that tinkering with it or putting it into the chest of another person was deeply, spiritually wrong. To him, it was spiritually wrong to withhold life-saving treatments. On this point, Kantrowitz agreed: "You know, the heart . . . people say it's the seat of the soul, or the organ of love," he said. "I don't know much about the soul, and as for love, there are better organs for that. No, it's a pump."

Kantrowitz, as well as Norman Shumway at Stanford, was already experimenting with heart transplants in animals, but Cooley and other surgeons knew there was a legal issue to be resolved before any heart was transplanted between human beings. The legal and medical definition of death at that time included the lack of a heartbeat. But when it came to transplanting a heart from one person to another, a non-beating heart was useless. Death itself had to be redefined before doctors could start transplanting hearts. If, for instance, a lack of brain activity could also be used to define death, then Cooley would head for the operating room free and clear. Until then, he was stuck.

Waiting was not Cooley's strong suit. He distracted himself with another big idea: a hospital devoted entirely and exclusively to solving the myriad problems caused by heart disease. Raising money from his Houston pals wasn't likely to be a problem. That kind of hospital would be a surefire moneymaker, given the prevalence of heart problems. At St. Luke's, Cooley was already doing three or four times as many surgeries as Methodist was doing, saving lives and throwing off cash like those early Texas gushers. But something else was eating at him: Cooley had heard that DeBakey was planning to build a special cardiovascular unit of his own, without including him.

In fact, DeBakey was on his way. He wasn't impressed with Cooley's access to the fortunes of rich Houstonians—DeBakey had tapped them too. That's how he got Methodist Hospital built as a showplace. But there wasn't much reason to go begging when he had access to millions for Baylor research projects from the National Institutes of Health.

Transplantation, however, was not high on DeBakey's list. Like Cooley, he had seen that the mere suggestion of the surgery inspired all kinds of public hysteria, and he wanted nothing to do with settling such ridiculous questions.

Besides, he was already under pressure on another front. De-Bakey's image had appeared on the cover of *Time* in 1965 with the headline "Toward an Artificial Heart." But now the man who had promised a mechanical heart to Congress in 1963 had become diverted by another idea: a "half heart" that would assist the left side of the heart. After all, most of the action was there: the left ventricle did all the heavy lifting, pumping blood to the rest of the body. (The right side is responsible only for pumping blood to the lungs.)

Like Kantrowitz, DeBakey was following a small body of new research that suggested a damaged heart could eventually return to normal with proper care. In July 1963, for instance, DeBakey's associate and Bud's mentor, Stanley Crawford, implanted a device designed to assist the pumping action of a damaged left ventricle; the patient lived for four days, enough time to incentivize the inventors, who declared the surgery a success because the pump was not the cause of death. "The pump was still working when he expired," noted DeBakey associate Domingo Liotta, who had devised the machine.

DeBakey also used federal grants to establish a joint task force with Rice University, located just across Main Street from the medical center. Rice engineers were then known to be some of the best in the world; they worked in the oil fields, and, in the early sixties, as the space program flourished, at NASA. This new team upped the weirdness factor in the labs—Rice engineers were known to be very smart but somewhat limited in social terms. These were the guys who seemed to have been born wearing pocket protectors.

For the next three years, this team continued its work on what they called a left ventricular assist device, LVAD for short. They didn't have much luck. DeBakey tried eight surgeries, and only two patients survived. (No doubt this pleased Team Cooley, who liked to claim that DeBakey was just too slow in the operating room. Heart surgery was a young man's game, and he was in his fifties.)

Then, in August 1966, DeBakey's team put an LVAD into a tiny thirty-seven-year-old woman from Mexico. She'd had rheumatic fever as a child and had been declining with heart disease for five years. By that point, she was spending most days in bed. But not only did Esperanza del Valle Vasquez survive the surgery; she also began to thrive. In just over a year, she was back at work in her Mexico City beauty parlor. Esperanza—the name means "hope" in Spanish—would live another six years, her life ending prematurely not because her heart failed but because of an auto accident. A widely disseminated photo—courtesy of Team DeBakey—shows Vasquez very much alive post-op, with tubes from the LVAD dangling just below her collarbone; her smile is radiant as she grasps DeBakey's hand and gazes worshipfully into his eyes. Soon after, Baylor signed contracts with a Los Angeles company for the manufacture of sixty-two LVADs.

Advantage, DeBakey. The editors at *Life* magazine—a masthead full of middle-aged white men who had or surely were developing heart problems themselves—were desperate for exclusives with the great doctor. (It didn't hurt DeBakey's press that he made a habit of meeting reporters in blood-spattered scrubs.) Though Houston cardiologists were quietly sending their patients to younger DeBakey associates like Stanley Crawford and George Noon, DeBakey's patient roster was packed with the rich and famous—from out of town.

But then something happened thousands of miles away, on the other side of the world. On December 4, 1967, a Cape Town surgeon by the name of Christiaan Barnard took the heart of a brain-dead young woman who had been hit by a car and sewed it into the chest of a fifty-five-year-old man named Louis Waskansky, who lived an astounding eighteen days.

Long before the age of social media, this news rocketed around the world, making headlines, interrupting television programs. It didn't hurt that Barnard was made for television: he had the twinkling blue eyes, the broad, sparkling smile, and the quick, seductive wit of a seasoned pol or a Hollywood star—yet another heart surgeon who gave healthy women palpitations. And now *he* was the hippest, hottest heart surgeon on earth. Unlike his colleagues in America, Barnard had not been hamstrung by silly laws about death determination, or any dithering about the spiritual qualities of the heart.

He had just gone and done it.

THE PURLOINED HEART

Today, heart transplants seem almost as routine as hip replacements. Anyone invited to observe transplant surgery at the Texas Heart Institute, for instance, would notice that Bud operated with all the drama of a dentist doing an annual cleaning. Ordinarily, the procedure takes around four hours—far less time than it takes to fly from New York to Paris. Hospital stays last about two weeks. The total cost ranges from $780,000 to close to $1 million, but, of course, very few people pay out of pocket. Medicare chips in, and most hospitals happily offer any number of plans to help a patient finance a new heart.

Even so, there is always a moment or two during surgery that would remind even the most jaded soul—at least, one who isn't a surgeon—that something pretty profound is going on. The first occurs after the patient has been laid out on the operating table and his body draped in paper; the only flesh visible is the chest, stained a brilliant yellow from the antibiotic wash. There aren't that many people in the room: a couple of docs, a few nurses, the perfusionist who connects the patient to the heart-lung machine, and the anesthesiologist, who makes sure he stays under and stays alive.

Then a surgeon—sometimes a younger associate—opens the chest, so as not to waste the time of the higher-priced expert, like Bud, who will do the real work. He makes the incision, cutting through tissue and muscle, pulls open the ribs with a retractor, and there it is: the heart, a spectrum of the most vivid shades of brown, red, yellow, and the palest blue, beating in its lair, bobbing on a tide of blood. If the heart is diseased, it might beat more faintly, or it might be covered by a layer of bright yellow fat, or it might be supersized because it's grown too large with muscle trying to compensate for its inability to pump enough blood.

Still, it is a living heart—that is, until the operator of the heart-lung machine flips a couple of switches and the machine takes over its business. (Today, the bypass machine is about the size of a small central air-conditioning unit on wheels, with myriad dials and gauges, along with tubes and vats for circulating and oxygenating the blood.) Once that happens, the heartbeat slows and then finally stops.

Enter Bud Frazier. He wears tired pale green scrubs with one of his even more tired burnt-orange UT Longhorn T-shirts underneath. Strands of curly white hair resist the confines of his surgical cap, and there are bright lights attached to the rims of his operating glasses. He leans over the patient and starts clipping away with his big, football player's hands until he reaches familiar terrain. He cuts the heart loose from its moorings. Then he lifts it out and hands it to a nurse who readies it for the pathology lab with about as much ceremony as a beleaguered husband taking out the trash. Bud has already turned back to the patient on the table, who now has an empty cavity that to a layperson might appear as dark and infinite as outer space, but to the surgeon just represents intermission.

Next, a nurse reaches into a Styrofoam cooler—the kind you would take on a picnic—and pulls out the new heart, which has been wrapped in plastic and packed in ice. She hands it over. Maybe it came from someone who died in a car accident, or a knife fight, or some other horrible fluke that causes grief to his or her family and a compromised joy for the recipient. The heart is a little pale from lack of circulation. That paleness contrasts with Bud's gloves, bright blue and now flecked with red blood turning brown in spots where it's dried. He takes the heart in his hands and eases it into the empty space, and then keeps pushing and prodding with some force, until he likes the position. Then he goes to work, sewing the donor heart in place, connecting it to the pulmonary artery and the aorta, and the atria—the circulatory system's main entrances and exits.

Finished, Bud stands back for a minute and waits; so does everyone else in the room except for the perfusionist, who is busy with his dials and switches again. He is the only person who isn't staring at the chest of the patient. He's weaning the patient off the machine.

And then it happens: the new heart begins to take on a richer color as it fills with blood. It begins to beat, searching for and then finding a normal rhythm, settling into its new home. The associate steps in again to close up the chest. Bud exits, snaps off his gloves, unties his gown and cap, pushes a hand through his hair, and goes back to his office, where he checks his messages, watches a little on Turner Classic Movies, or, maybe, takes a nap.

Bud has never believed a heart transplant to be a cure-all. He will tell you that a person is really just exchanging one set of medical problems for another. Pain gets traded for medication and constant monitoring, though you get the chance to walk around the block, go out to dinner, or on a good day hit the mall. As a younger surgeon, Bud had been skeptical of the value. But now his son and daughter have children of their own, and the idea that his kids' lives could be cut short—that they wouldn't live to see their kids grow up, as he has—is something he prefers not to imagine.

—∿—

Bud was rescuing wounded boys from Central Highlands mountainsides when Christiaan Barnard performed the first human heart transplant. Some years earlier, Barnard had come through Houston for some training with DeBakey, but, the story goes, no one had been particularly impressed with his abilities. (Getting heart surgeons to praise one another is like asking the same of trial lawyers. It rarely happens.) Now, as news of Barnard's success circled the globe, there was a lot of gnashing of teeth and rending of garments among the small community of American heart surgeons. In 1968, the concept of brain death was finally accepted in the United States, partly with the proof of flat brain waves provided by the EEG machine, but thanks also to ratification of a definition by the 22nd World Medical Assembly, and by an article that appeared defining irreversible comas in the *Journal of the American Medical Association* by a group from Harvard Medical School that may or may not have been influenced by Barnard's triumph.

Anticipating the official go-ahead, Shumway at Stanford and Kantrowitz in New York had been racing each other to be the first to transplant a heart, and were caught flat-footed by the events in South Africa. Cooley wasn't happy about it either. He sent Barnard a telegram: "Congratulations on your first transplant, Chris. I will be reporting my first hundred soon." But it was Kantrowitz who crossed the finish line next by transplanting a heart from an eighteen-day-old baby into one who was two days old—and died within hours.

The biggest surprise—after Barnard's success—was DeBakey's reaction. He had been skeptical of transplantation because of all the sociological problems it caused—and because he had spent years publicly and privately touting mechanical replacements for the heart. Now he made a hairpin turn and swiftly organized a transplant committee at Baylor. Once again he snubbed Cooley, even though Cooley was still a prominent member of the medical school faculty and even though he was, and not solely by his own admission, a leader in the field. (In 1967, for instance, the International Surgical Society gave Cooley its highest honor and called him "the most valuable surgeon of the heart and blood vessel anywhere in the world.")

"Maybe it's immodest of me," Cooley wrote in his autobiography, "but I thought that since I was the most experienced heart surgeon in the world, I was the one best qualified to perform transplants in Houston."

Still, DeBakey's snub left Cooley free to proceed on his own. His Texas Heart Institute had fast become a reality. Ground had been broken in 1967 on a building connected to St. Luke's Hospital, a contemporary high-rise of coffee-colored brick well stocked with state-of-the-art operating rooms. (Some would have glass-domed ceilings, so that visitors on the floor above could watch the surgeries.) Yet another grateful Cooley patient from the oil business had donated the initial $5 million, with more flowing in from other locals as well as thankful patients from around the globe. Now Cooley didn't have to fight DeBakey for beds or funds. ("Denton just got tired of sucking hind tit," was the way one colleague put it.) He was where he most liked to be: in the land of the free.

But now he had been beaten by a South African surgeon with half his talent. It was untenable.

—⋀⋀—

Cooley nursed his injured pride for six miserable months until, in May 1968, he saw his chance in the form of Everett Thomas, who was wasting away in a hospital bed at St. Luke's. Thomas was only forty-seven but had suffered two strokes and two heart attacks. It was clear—to Cooley, at least—that a transplant was Thomas' only option. It was fortuitous, then, that a fifteen-year-old girl shot herself in the face after arguing with her nineteen-year-old husband, and arrived at St. Luke's with flat brain waves. Two Cooley associates talked with her parents, who gave permission to donate her heart. It might not have been much of a discussion: Cooley had operated on the poor girl to correct a congenital defect a decade or so before.

Cooley, who was speaking at a medical conference in Louisiana, raced back to Houston on a chartered plane and immediately set up two operating rooms, one for the donor and one for the recipient. He figured that transplanting a heart would be easy, even if he hadn't done it before. Certainly it would be easier than the tedious, intricate operations he was doing almost daily on the tiny diseased hearts of children. All he had to do was cut out Thomas' damaged heart and sew in the new one. Then he would unhook the clamps, let the blood pour into the new heart, and, presto, Everett Thomas would be a new man.

When he got into the operating room, Cooley as always worked intuitively, which was just about his only choice. He knew his destination, but there were no maps to show him how to get there. He had a moment of doubt when he removed the vascular clamps and the heart started—but with an irregular beat. Cooley turned to the nurse holding the defibrillator paddles and grabbed them out of her hands, pressing them into Thomas' chest to give his heart a shock. There was a buzz as electricity traveled from the paddles to the heart, then silence. Cooley stared down at the new heart, willing it to perform. Now it was he, not Thomas, who was barely breathing.

Seconds passed, and then . . . damned if Thomas' heart didn't begin to beat normally, as if it had finally caught the melody of a familiar tune. Cooley had done in thirty-five minutes what had taken Barnard nine hours.

Now it was Cooley's turn to be the international sensation—again. He could now claim that he had completed the first *success-*

ful heart transplant in the United States, because Thomas—unlike Barnard and Kantrowitz's poor souls—was alive and well. Reporters raced to the hospital; one even suffered a broken leg in the crush to get to a press conference. Then came the desperate, in droves. One got to Houston on a jet provided by his congressman. A man from Kentucky demanded Cooley give him a penis transplant. The "waiters," as they were called, fought for a room in the already packed motels ringing the Texas Medical Center, letting their hopes take flight every time an ambulance pulled into St. Luke's emergency entrance with its sirens blazing. Cooley didn't mind the death threats he got from those who believed that transplanting a heart was against the will of God. He was back on top. And he'd heard that when De-Bakey got the news, he had canceled his surgeries for the day and locked himself in his office.

The truth was, DeBakey had been dragging his heels with his own transplant team. Finally the Methodist surgeons, desperate to keep up, had to push their chief to make a move. In particular, a talented and ambitious surgeon by the name of Ted Dietrich, who had long been studying the possibility of multiple organ transplants, urged DeBakey to join the march of progress—or be trampled into the dust of obscurity. In fact, they had to do better, which was why, three or so months after Cooley's triumph, Dietrich and DeBakey went into their operating room and transplanted not just a heart but a lung and both kidneys.

Cooley countered by taking the ever-so-tiny heart and lungs from a brain-dead baby and sewing them into the chest of a two-month-old. The child died fourteen hours later, but in this new, miraculous world of transplantation, the operation was still considered a success. You could build on fourteen hours.

By the end of 1968, there was only one place to go for a heart transplant: Houston, Texas. Cooley had performed seventeen of them, more than anyone in the world. Along with DeBakey, he was now also among the richest surgeons in the world—easily a multimillionaire—and he had turned the Texas Heart Institute into a mecca not just for patients but also for doctors who wanted to learn at the feet of the master.

That was the good news. The bad news was that by the end of that year, only four of DeBakey's ten transplanted patients and three of Cooley's were still alive. Everett Thomas, who was tethered to the hospital for so long that Cooley had found him a job as a trust officer at a nearby bank, died after seven months, the longest survivor. Other surgeons around the world were reporting similar failure rates, and had started talking about a moratorium on transplants, first privately and then publicly. It was commonly believed the patients were dying of rejection—their bodies wouldn't accept the heart of another human. No one knew why. Maybe the whole thing had been a crazy idea from the start.

Many in the press thought that way. "Transplants, Apollo Both Misguided?" asked a story by Judith Randal in the *Washington Star* in 1969. "Many people see, in the proliferation of heart transplants and in the space race, efforts to keep up with the Joneses rather than a concern for doing our own thing." The story went on to suggest that most Americans would prefer a cure from cancer over a Mars landing.

Meanwhile, Cooley saw that with every death, the public was becoming less and less willing to donate their own hearts or those of their loved ones. He knew that the drop-off in donors would mean they would never be able to understand what was going wrong. Hoping to change minds, he starred in a television commercial for the Living Bank and declared his own willingness to be a donor. But nothing helped. "I can respect, if not agree with, the contention of some people that the spirit or the soul or what have you resides in the heart," he would write. "But it was impossible for me to in any way agree with those otherwise enlightened people who chose to relegate the viable organs of their loved ones to dust when those same organs would have provided hope for people who were dying in wait. It was frustrating as hell."

—⟋⟍⟋⟍—

Cooley brooded in his private office, the one conveniently situated among his six operating rooms. It was a cramped, spare place, probably because Louise Cooley hadn't applied her decorating skills as she had upstairs, in her husband's baronial public suite. Down here, it was that pinkish-green fluorescent lighting that set off the photo of his transplant team with a quote from André Gide: "Man cannot discover new oceans unless he has the courage to lose sight of the shore." Cooley, now forty-eight, was stymied, a feeling he ranked alongside introspection on the scale of useless mental states. A different kind of man would have been distracted by all the turmoil that had taken place outside the hospital in 1968—the race riots, the ongoing Vietnam War, the assassinations of Martin Luther King Jr. and Robert F. Kennedy, the student protests around the world, the beginnings of the women's movement, the Soviet invasion of Czechoslovakia, Jacqueline Kennedy's traitorous marriage to Greek shipping magnate Aristotle Onassis. But Cooley wasn't drawn to dinner-table debates. He was a Nixon man. He believed in the war in Vietnam. He saw no parallels in the rebelliousness that was sweeping the United States and the powerful internal pressure that pushed him to go his own way. Hippies in Haight-Ashbury? He grew his sideburns a little longer, that was it.

The only event that did galvanize Cooley was the proposed launch of Apollo 8 in December. American astronauts, running second to the Soviets, were finally going to orbit the moon—just as Kennedy had pledged in 1962. But Cooley knew better than most that DeBakey's simultaneous promise to eradicate heart disease with a mechanical heart was going nowhere. Cooley knew this because he knew his nemesis. Mike DeBakey wasn't a risk taker.

Then, on a sweltering day in July, Cooley was replacing an aortic valve on a middle-aged man when the man developed "stone heart," a rigor-mortis-like condition when an already damaged heart literally begins to harden and die in the surgeon's hands. Everyone in the room understood. The look of defeat could be seen in their eyes, visible between their caps and masks. No donor heart was waiting in an ice chest nearby, and there certainly wasn't time to retrieve one, assuming one could even be found. And, of course, no artificial heart existed that could keep the patient alive until a real replacement could be transplanted. Cooley's patient had run out of options, and so had he.

But Cooley, his gloves coated crimson, wouldn't stop. He had one last idea; he ordered an associate to the lab, who returned with an anesthetized sheep, ready for surgery. In an adjacent operating room, they cut out the animal's heart, and soon enough Cooley was sewing it into his patient before anyone in the room could really fathom what was happening.

In 1969, there were no plaintiff's lawyers squatting in the hospital lobby, no rules guiding what a surgeon could or could not do in an emergency. As Cooley saw it, his job was to save lives. If the sheep's heart lasted even a few hours, maybe he could find a human heart donor, and a crazy idea wouldn't seem so crazy.

Finished, Cooley plucked off the clamps and waited for the blood to start flowing into the heart, causing it to turn that familiar, robust pink. Instead . . . nothing. The sheep's heart shrank and then shriveled, and Cooley could do nothing but watch his patient go.

A few months later, he told a group of reporters that he had begun to work on an artificial heart.

The only problem was, Cooley didn't have one. He just had an *idea* of one. The person who actually had an artificial heart was Domingo Liotta, who had been working on his own while DeBakey pushed for the heart assist devices—the LVADs—in the Baylor lab. A taciturn, somewhat dour man in public, Liotta was privately a bit on the baroque side, especially when he took to the page. As Liotta would later write of Cooley's sudden interest, it was "not needful to express my full conviction of this wisdom."

In fact, Liotta was feeling like a jilted lover. Initially, the great Michael DeBakey had been willing to do anything for the researcher he had enticed from Willem Kolff's lab, the Argentine immigrant who was certain he could build an artificial heart. DeBakey eased Liotta's visa woes and ordered any equipment Liotta desired. He got Liotta an appointment as an advanced research fellow in cardiac surgery through the American Heart Association, which doubled his pay. DeBakey even stonewalled the dean of the medical school back in Argentina, who wanted Liotta back. His presence in Houston was crucial to medical progress, DeBakey insisted.

But gradually DeBakey seemed to lose interest in Liotta and his grand plan. The more work they did, the more DeBakey saw that he had profoundly underestimated the complexity of the heart and the biomedical challenges of building a successful replacement. In fact, these were problems that would remain for decades to come. The main issue was with the blood, which, like the heart, had a particular way of doing things. If an artificial heart couldn't push the blood through the body evenly and fast enough, it would pool and form clots, eventually blocking pathways and causing a stroke. But if a pump pushed blood through the body too fast, its delicate red blood cells would break up from the stress, depleting the blood of crucial oxygen. This too could be fatal.

Once Liotta started implanting his device in calves, DeBakey became even less interested. The heart was made of hard plastic and was about the size of a honeydew melon, with two chambers; they looked a little like two flattened-out versions of the planet Saturn. An air compressor about the size of an upright piano was supposed to power the pumping action. But it just didn't work very well: out of seven calves, only one lived—for forty-four hours. DeBakey got a look and described the lone survivor as "a cadaver from time of implantation." So it wasn't very surprising that DeBakey started backpedaling on the total heart he had once promised would be ready by 1969. Now, he said, it looked more like 1972. Or maybe 1973.

Then too, President Richard Nixon didn't share his predecessors' passion for a high-tech war on heart disease. Prevention was becoming the new buzzword—maybe the government should be urging people to eat less, smoke less, and exercise more instead of funding weird experimental devices. Besides, prevention was a lot cheaper.

DeBakey, with the distant early warning system of a bat, decided to focus solely on the left ventricular assist device, which, after all, had worked at least once: on Esperanza del Valle, the grateful hairdresser from Mexico. He had spent the following year implanting a few more, with mixed results—though as time went on, the LVAD experiments looked a lot more promising than heart transplants.

Ditto the total artificial heart. Yes, DeBakey had hired Liotta to work on one, but now he ordered Liotta to work exclusively on LVADs. When Liotta tried to complain, DeBakey refused to return his phone calls or answer his memos; when Liotta showed DeBakey a model of an artificial heart he was refining, DeBakey, exasperated, demanded Liotta put it away and never show it to him again. After all, he was busy running Baylor—DeBakey consolidated his power by becoming president in 1968—and lecturing around the globe, *and* providing comment to newspapers and television programs, *and* tending to his own surgical practice, *and* proofing the articles his sisters wrote under his name for journals. He never seemed to sleep, and neither did his sisters, who kept the DeBakey grandeur machine functioning a lot more effectively than Liotta's phony heart.

Liotta licked his wounds and, in secret, convinced a few members of DeBakey's team to improve on his prototype. By September 1968, he had one—but not for DeBakey. At some point after Cooley's unfortunate sheep heart transplant (for which Liotta had been present), he and Cooley had started talking about a collaboration. Cooley had listened to Liotta's complaints, and attributed the failure of Liotta's artificial heart in the calves to DeBakey's slowness as a surgeon. With the help of a new team, he and Liotta agreed to work on a heart of their own. They came up with something . . . much like the original.

That both Cooley and Liotta were members of the Baylor faculty and that Liotta's device had been developed at Baylor with a National Heart Institute grant wasn't troubling to them. Of *course* they would have to fabricate a new heart and a new console so that this heart wouldn't be confused with the Baylor heart. And it was understood that the device would be used *only in an emergency* and *only temporarily,* until it could be replaced with a human heart. "Neither of us felt a need to ask Mike's permission to proceed," Cooley explained later. "After all, he'd already said that he wanted Domingo to work on the LVAD project." More to the point, Cooley and Liotta were required to submit their plan to a Baylor committee for approval, a committee DeBakey ran. His history of previous denials suggested to Cooley that he would turn this project down as well. So Cooley and Liotta came to the mutual decision that it would be better to ask for forgiveness than permission. Or, as Liotta would write in his memoir: "Cooley and I moved forward in the accomplishment of the risky decision . . . venturing under the influence of the clear and always fascinating summons of medicine. We disregarded our already renowned careers and paid no attention to the threatening surroundings that were growing at the University."

—∿—

The Illinois couple who collided with Cooley's new plan were named Shirley and Haskell Karp. Haskell, forty-seven, was a man of very modest means—at home in Skokie, he worked in a print shop as the price estimator, while Shirley was a homemaker and mother to their three young sons. Haskell was quiet and wry behind his horn-rimmed glasses; she was wide-eyed, raven-haired, and a little high-strung. They had come to the Texas Heart Institute in desperation, like so many of Cooley's patients—other doctors had sent Haskell home to die. His heart was so weak and damaged that it could stop beating at any minute.

Cooley saw things differently. He had a voice that was both soft and hard, a homey Texas accent that, combined with his radiant confidence, could almost always make bad news a little easier to take. Haskell, he told the couple, had an aneurysm on the left ventricle that was one source of damage; another was destruction of heart muscle from previous heart attacks. The solution was simple. "What you need is a new heart!" Cooley announced. He promised to try to repair the heart first, but if he couldn't, a transplant was the only option. To keep Karp alive until he could find a donor, he had a new device he could try, something that could tide Haskell over at least until he could find the human heart to replace it with. Something that would serve as a bridge to transplant—a bridge heart, kind of like a bridge loan. The Karps signed the release Cooley gave them. They were hopeful.

On April 4, 1969, Haskell was wheeled into the operating room. Cooley opened his chest, got a good look at the left and right ventricles, and knew right away that this patient's was the worst-looking heart he'd ever seen. The inside wall was covered in scar tissue. It reminded Cooley of a battered, deflated basketball. He cut away as much scar tissue as he could, hoping that repair would save the heart, but then there wasn't enough left to function. When Cooley released the clamps, he got blood flow, but only a faint, irregular heartbeat. Electric shocks and manual massage did no good, and neither did an injection of drugs. Haskell Karp was going to die, probably in the next few minutes.

Cooley had to make a decision: to let his patient go or to try Liotta's artificial heart. Quietly he asked that the device and the console be brought in, while he started cutting out what remained of Haskell's heart. "Have St. Luke's and Mrs. Karp ask for a donor as soon as possible," he ordered. Scour the country, stat.

The operating room, so silent and grim, now sprang to life. Someone wheeled in the command console. A scrub nurse came in bearing a steel bowl in both hands, like an offering. Inside was something white and translucent, with small cuffs blossoming at the top and connections for tubes extending from the bottom. No one noticed when Cooley's secretary tiptoed out of the observation gallery. Her pace quickened to a trot and then a run as she headed for St. Luke's public relations department, to tell them that Cooley was implanting an artificial heart for the first time in history.

Even for a surgeon as gifted as Cooley, the implantation didn't go easily. The device was stiff, and the material used on the cuffs designed as connectors from human muscle to plastic kept blunting the needle where he tried to sew it in. Cooley worked intently on one side at a time, stitching the left atrium of Karp's heart to the corresponding artificial side. Then he did the same on the right. Then he threaded the two narrow plastic drive lines that pumped pressurized carbon dioxide under the skin, through the heart cavity, down through the abdomen, and into the console.

"Okay, Domingo, let's see how well this thing works in a human being," Cooley said, standing back for the first time in hours. A technician flipped a switch, and within a few seconds a reddish cast became visible inside the plastic. Blood was flowing toward the mechanical heart. A few people began to whisper prayers. Liotta thought the time was right: he ordered the operator of the heart-lung machine to start weaning Karp off the pump. After a few minutes, Cooley told him to stop entirely. The surgery had taken forty-seven minutes, but Karp had been on the pump for a risky two hours. No one knew whether he would make it or not, and if he did, what condition he would be in.

But then Karp's new heart began to work. His chest began to rise and fall on its own. It seemed then as if he was breathing for everyone in the operating room.

Within fifteen minutes after Cooley had closed his chest, Karp was conscious, able to move his fingers and toes on command. His organs appeared to be functioning normally.

For once, Cooley could not maintain his composure. With damp eyes, he shook the hand of the man operating the power console, and then found Liotta. Liotta would recall Cooley's words to him for the rest of his life, though maybe something was lost in the translation: "Domingo, we administered to Baylor University the biggest enema; it will be remembered in years to come."

EXPERIMENTS

One of Bud Frazier's most beloved spots on earth sits five floors below his book-strewn office and two floors below ground level inside St. Luke's and the Texas Heart Institute. To get there requires a change of elevators—only one goes to the second basement—and a mastery of the hospital's nearly indecipherable maze of color-coded hallways. The door to this place is always locked, and anyone who makes it through has to sign in. This is the THI's research lab. Cooley put Bud in charge of it in 1981.

It's the kind of place that would make a PETA volunteer apoplectic, one reason its location remains, if not secret, at least unadvertised. Science isn't always pretty, metaphorically or literally. The only light here comes from the grayish white of fluorescent tubes. The walls are an institutional green; along with two spacious operating rooms, there are calves and goats and sheep and pigs, some sleeping and grunting in pens, some hooked up to tubes and monitors and held in place in what resemble milking stanchions. To the uninitiated, it does look like an undesignated circle of animal hell, but of course that is not how the people who work there see the place, because they have seen the results of the animal sacrifices: at best—though not always, because failure is such a regular occurrence—patients lived because they died. The lab is living proof of science and medicine at one of the most painful crossroads.

For Bud, the lab is a sanctuary—"the best in the world," he is prone to say, even though it might have some competition after some forty-plus years. But it is indisputably the scene of four decades of disasters and triumphs in the war against heart disease, especially when it comes to implanted devices. Maybe for this reason, Bud shows a mournful gratitude toward the animals here, especially the calves, who remind him of his childhood in West Texas. "They are sweet animals," he says wistfully, positioning himself by a stanchion and scratching the ears of some doomed bovine.

When Bud returned to the Texas Medical Center to finish the residency the draft and the Vietnam War had so rudely interrupted, he found himself in the middle of the escalating war between De-Bakey and Cooley.

DeBakey had learned about the Karp surgery like just about everyone else. On April 4, 1969—the day of the operation—he had flown to Washington for a meeting with fellow members of the Artificial Heart Myocardial Infarction Advisory Committee of the National Heart Institute. Though there are some rumors he might have been tipped off that night, DeBakey's own account reports that he was alerted the next morning at the meeting, when members of the committee surrounded him. They had read about this great cardiac leap forward in the papers or heard about it on the news. They couldn't wait to talk about it! DeBakey listened—desperate to hide his shock, no doubt—and realized that the heart Cooley had used "was similar to that which we had developed in our laboratories." On purpose or by accident, Denton Cooley had found a brilliant way to embarrass his nemesis: in front of his peers.

Once DeBakey returned home, he fired virtually everyone in the lab, added more locks to his office doors, and appeared to have given up on the creation of a total artificial heart. A period of cardiac repair stasis set in at Methodist. Meanwhile, Cooley was turning the Texas Heart Institute—literally a stone's throw to the south—into a heart surgery colossus. Bud had missed the Karp episode in its entirety, and so maybe underestimated its importance. He arranged to work at THI after finishing his general surgery residency. He wanted to specialize in cardiothoracic surgery, and do more research on heart support devices.

It did not occur to him that a simple transfer would be perceived by DeBakey as a betrayal on the scale of Benedict Arnold's. But once DeBakey got word that Bud was intending to move to the Cooley camp—no matter what his reasons or his future intentions— DeBakey cut him dead. Even Bud's kindhearted mentor Stanley Crawford would scoot away when Bud approached, afraid that De- Bakey would fire him for being seen anywhere close to Frazier the Traitor.

On the upside, Bud soon found he had moved from a capricious dictatorship to an elite fraternity. The Texas Heart Institute at that time was like no other institution in the world. If DeBakey was a brilliant manipulator of the vastly expanding medical/governmental complex, Cooley was someone who gave the appearance of bucking it at every turn. Thanks to the continued rise in heart disease, the breathless media coverage of potential surgical cures in the likes of *Time* and *Life* magazines, and a declining public interest in space after the moon landing in 1969, heart surgeons were gaining on the astronauts as the new American heroes. The problem was, most heart surgeons didn't look or act like the astronauts. DeBakey was no one's idea of a cover boy, and neither were Adrian Kantrowitz in New York and Norman Shumway at Stanford.

But Cooley was good looking and soft-spoken, with a veneer of shyness that gave cover to his voracious ambition. ("A successful cardiovascular surgeon should be a man who, when asked to name the three best surgeons in the world, would have difficulty deciding the other two," he once said.) He embodied certain mythic characteristics thought to be deeply embedded in the American DNA, qualities that were even more pronounced in the Texas archetype—independence, individualism, and self-determination. Then too, Cooley had no aversion to making a lot of money. DeBakey had to run a medical school and ride herd on a hospital while attending to his own patients, while speaking worldwide and racing back and forth to influence policy in Washington. Cooley was learning to love the limelight—he met the Pope at a well-publicized meeting in 1969—but he loved building THI more. And he loved performing the diciest, most demanding heart surgeries more than that. Sure, there were other stars in the firmament, but to play on Cooley's team meant not only that you were fighting on the front lines against heart disease but also that you had the freedom to operate, literally and metaphorically, without constraints.

And you had an endless supply of patients. The heist—though Cooley didn't call it that—of the Liotta heart had not hurt Cooley's reputation with patients, even if it caused consternation among his peers. By the early 1970s, a seemingly infinite stream of heart patients were flooding into the Texas Heart Institute every day, clamoring to be saved; forty-six hundred people had heart surgery at THI in 1974. Like DeBakey, Cooley's patients came from up and down the economic spectrum and from all parts of the world—a little girl from Vietnam; the Iranian prime minister's deputy chief; Zeppo Marx; Hall of Fame Yankee pitcher Whitey Ford; and so on. Patients arrived by private plane from the Middle East, or by airlifts courtesy of the Dutch government, or by pickup truck from some innocuous blue-collar suburb of Houston. Cooley became a favorite surgeon of a roving band of genuine Gypsies, who never seemed to leave the hospital without taking something that wasn't theirs. Bud kept a copy of a *Houston Chronicle* classified ad for a heart-lung machine, assuming they had been the culprits.

The US government flew in poor kids from all over the country. Not for nothing had Cooley cultivated the Heart Institute's affiliation with Texas Children's Hospital next door when he'd been a Baylor professor. Both heart surgery and his own career had had its beginnings with previously impossible operations on children; now, no one was better at operating on the smallest hearts than he.

For all these reasons, Denton Cooley was not only world-famous but rich beyond his wildest imaginings. Free of Baylor, he no longer had to donate a portion of his earnings to the school, as DeBakey required. A multimillionaire when it meant something to be one, Cooley was now richer than even some of his wildcatter buddies. To his colonnaded, antebellum-style mansion in River Oaks and his Cool Acres ranch on the Brazos, he added a house in Galveston, and a "ski shack" on the San Jacinto River where he took Christiaan Barnard waterskiing. He gave tours of THI to the aged Charles Lindbergh. Louise Cooley became a regular on the social scene and in the society pages. With her husband so often occupied at the hospital, her walker was the society hairdresser of that day, whose name was, yes, Lyndon Johnson. Partly because Cooley was busy and partly because he was famously cheap, family vacations often happened in tandem with speaking engagements and honorary events, like meeting the Pope.

But Cooley couldn't operate on everyone—forty cases were a daily average for his team; one day Cooley did fourteen alone, "and they were all tough cases," Bud noted. A gifted surgeon elsewhere might do one tough case and two easy ones, in comparison. To be one of Cooley's chosen associates, then, was equal to being a knight of the Round Table. Cooley was unquestionably their chief. He never seemed to lose his temper. If he was disappointed in a surgeon's work, he just became more distant. But you had to keep up. "Cooley didn't teach you anything but you learned a lot," Bud often said. He was the kind of leader who simply assumed that others would do what was expected, and in large part they did, his associates evolving from a team of acolytes into something more akin to a restless, ambitious group of young men determined to make their own reputations in the wake of their leader.

This was possible because Cooley set up assembly-line surgery at THI. There were eight operating rooms designed around a central pod where other surgeons opened and closed for him, and where, given the teeming census, one of Cooley's chosen might perform an actual valve repair or coronary bypass while Cooley himself worked on a more difficult case next door. So an associate could wind up doing almost as much surgery as the great man himself, perfecting his skills and publishing his own discoveries while enhancing the status of THI and Houston too.

The space program may have been providing less inspiration in Houston as it shifted toward the humdrum shuttle voyages by the late seventies and early eighties, but the oil boom was on. In an interesting and fortuitous (for surgeons) series of coincidences, the stress of success—and then failure, when the dreaded oil bust of the mid-eighties set in—made for still more surgeries and still more donations from grateful patients. It was a badge of honor to have Denton Cooley's home number in your personal phone book. Even more prestigious to recover—and then lose to him at golf.

But whatever the rewards, there was a price to be paid. The patients who came to the Texas Heart Institute in its earliest days were desperately ill, as were the children at Texas Children's Hospital next door. On Bud's first day, he watched Cooley reassure an angelic six-year-old girl that he would unzip her chest, fix her heart, and then zip her right up again. She never made it off the operating table, and neither did two other children that same day. "Today was a bad day," Cooley told his troops, "but tomorrow will be better."

So it was for all those reasons that Bud left his wife and two small children at home in the Montrose around five-thirty every morning and returned late at night. Sometimes he took his daughter, Allison, on early-morning rounds, the tiny girl with silky blond hair and stars in her eyes grasping her father's hand as they strode down the halls. Surgery dominated the Frazier family dinner conversations, with Bud spinning ongoing mealtime dramas from his life-and-death cases. But many times, Bud didn't make it home at all—Cooley and DeBakey had their differences, but superhuman endurance was the one thing they had in common. The 24/7 workweek was just as de rigueur at Texas Heart Institute as it had been at DeBakey's five-star, high-pressure Methodist Hospital.

Bud learned. He became a stellar transplant surgeon, but he was also the *only* surgeon at THI who volunteered for that particular duty in the early days. Most of his colleagues begged off: too many patients died, either waiting to get a heart, or while they were being operated on, or after they got one. They just couldn't take it. Bud could, for reasons he did not choose to examine. If he had done so, he might have examined his eagerness to please at all costs, his passion for virtuous sacrifice, and his boundless love for the action of the hospital, which was so much more dramatic and rewarding than ordinary life. Even if he was sleeping in his office instead of going to Todd's basketball game or going out for Mexican food with Rachel, Bud could be there, waiting for something to happen that might just challenge everything he had. He never had to ask whether he was doing good. He knew he was.

Once, after a couple of drinks on an airplane, he asked Cooley how he dealt with the pressures of being a surgeon, of losing patient after patient year in and year out. What was his secret, Bud wanted to know? Cooley looked at him squarely. "To kill with impunity," he deadpanned. Bud got the joke: you just got on with it. The failure of one save would eventually produce rescue somewhere else.

By the early 1980s, he was also reaping the enormous rewards bestowed on the heart surgeons of his day, especially those at the Texas Heart Institute. By that time, St. Luke's was doing more pump cases—heart surgeries with the heart-lung machine—than in all of Western Europe, 5,000 alone in 1981. Not only was Bud publishing papers in the most prestigious journals, he was invited to demonstrate his techniques in places like Russia and the Middle East. He spoke often at medical conferences that always seemed to be held in garden spots from Tahiti to Florence to Tokyo. He dined at a royal function in London with Princess Anne, and at another colloquium politely turned down a threesome with Christiaan Barnard and his beauty queen lover.

And Bud, like so many of his peers, developed an antipathy to being challenged. He could fight back with a fury that, in such a large man, could be intimidating, if not downright frightening. He once showed up at a deposition in DeBakey-style bloody scrubs. The lawyers cringed when Bud launched into what an attorney would later describe as an opening statement, something about Bud being the only person standing between the patient and God, and how dare they interrupt his work for something as insignificant as a lawsuit, and so on. In general, Bud fostered a deep and abiding antipathy to anyone who knew nothing about medicine but still felt it was fine to impinge on his dire day-to-day routine. Lawyers were at the top of his list.

The disagreements would become more frequent over the years, and were not just limited to lawyers. When patients begged Bud for their lives—and they did beg—he couldn't say no, no matter how risky or experimental the procedure. Wasn't THI's reputation that they treated the sickest of the sick? Hospital administrators worried that he was treating people who should have been allowed to die. Bud wouldn't hear of it. Forms, permissions? Those were for other people to worry about. His job was to save people. If the hospital wanted to help, they could give him more personnel in the operating room, which he asked for repeatedly. "As noted, we have no night coverage for transplants or LVADs," he would write one administrator. "I'm here at least two to three nights a week. . . . We are also the only hospital in the country without a [critical care specialist] in the ICU." Bud didn't worry about his numbers, the mortality statistics that were sometimes lower at St. Luke's than at places like Stanford or the Mayo Clinic. He argued that they didn't take the risks he did—they followed in his wake, once he had perfected a technique. He had a certainty and an authority the administrators lacked, and so they went along, even as medical costs were escalating, even if they disagreed. There were colleagues who warned Bud that he could wind up in political hot water. He ignored them too.

The only person Bud couldn't and wouldn't intimidate was, of course, Cooley. When Cooley was too cheap to pay for two rooms at a luxury hotel, Bud agreed to bunk with him and share the cost. When they were in Paris and dining at a very expensive restaurant with the mother of a patient—the actress Olivia de Havilland—Bud picked up the check after Cooley palmed it his way.

But Cooley did reward loyalty and ability, and by 1980 Bud found himself head of the institute's heart transplant program. If this seemed more like a punishment than a reward, times had changed—again. Barnard's triumph had been followed by the disasters of the late 1960s, when no one survived what had seemed at first to be an astounding medical breakthrough. No one knew then why the bodies of transplant recipients rejected the foreign organ, or why their immune systems kicked into high gear to fight it. The patients just died, sometimes sooner, sometimes later.

But then, in the early 1970s, a researcher at Sandoz, a multinational drug company, was looking for new uses of shelved drugs. One of those was a product called cyclosporine, which he thought might be used to help fungal infections. But when he gave the drug to mice, they got sicker instead—the drug was tamping down their immune systems. That was bad for the mice, but led to a new line of inquiry: what if the drug could be used to suppress the immune system, which would keep the body from fighting off a transplanted organ? By the early 1980s, doctors were trying it in liver and kidney transplants, and then with heart transplants. Patients lived; or, at least, survival rates increased from a few months to years, maybe even a decade. The miracle drug had literally brought the practice of heart transplantation back from the dead.

Bud saw its use with a twenty-four-year-old woman from Lubbock by the name of Rona Coleman. She had contracted postpartum cardiomyopathy, a rare form of heart failure that can occur after a woman gives birth. Coleman was so sick that her kidneys had stopped working, and she also had a terrible staph infection. Her skin had a ghastly yellow pallor. Her only option was a transplant, which she refused. In and out of consciousness, she managed to write Bud a note: "Let me die."

Bud talked to Coleman's husband, who put the decision in Bud's hands. Bud stalled, hoping a donor would appear. She had two children, along with the newborn, and a husband who loved her.

But then Coleman wrote Bud another note, asking him again to let her go. The nurses on the floor were so furious with Bud that they threatened to get a court order if he didn't agree to her wishes.

Then a heart magically appeared. Bud did the transplant, and, along with the usual meds and procedures, treated her with cyclosporine. Two months later, Rona Coleman was ready for hospital discharge.

"What do you think about the letters you sent me?" Bud asked her when he went to say his goodbyes.

She looked at him blankly. "What letters?" she asked.

The story became one Bud told over and over again, to interns and patients and friends and family. Few people understood how intently Bud believed in his mission to save his patients, how contemptuous he was of doctors who gave up too soon. He couldn't give up. Still, people died on his service every day, and they died even after he tried to save them every way he knew how.

Maybe that commitment was one reason Bud could never get too interested in the business side of his work. Other surgeons built hefty private practices; he just couldn't get his mind—or his psychology—around doing any such thing. He was rich enough. He didn't have the patience or the inclination to schmooze cardiologists for those all-important referrals. He was quickly bored at fundraising galas. He was an outlier. Yes, he wrote for prestigious cardiac journals, but he was happier reading dark Russian novels and Shakespearean tragedies, which were not exactly watercooler topics among his surgical colleagues in Houston. All told, it was natural that the THI lab became his refuge.

Like everything else at THI—and often in the Texas medical center—the lab wasn't really set up like other labs around the United States. In the sixties and seventies, Cooley saw research as a distraction from the thrill of surgery and its medical and financial rewards. "Cooley didn't care what you did," Bud liked to say. "If you could get paid for it, you could transplant heads." But on a plane coming back from a conference in Russia, he happened to meet a Harvard-trained African American surgeon by the name of John Norman who tutored him in the importance—for both medicine and fundraising—of research. By the time the plane landed, Cooley had cut a deal with Norman to come to THI and run the lab Liotta had started and never finished. As Cooley would later say of Norman, "I decided I needed this brilliant mind." Cooley wrangled $2 million from the oil-flush Cullen family for the lab, and Norman started in 1972.

It's easy to see how he was irresistible to Cooley: Norman had been deeply involved in experimental organ transplants—he and his team had used a pig's liver to keep a human patient alive for nearly three weeks. He had also been working on what were then called partial artificial hearts—what would come to be known as left ventricular assist devices, or LVADs. They were the coming thing: Richard Nixon had not been as entranced with total heart replacements as LBJ, and so the artificial heart program was being both scaled back and retooled.

Norman never made Houston home, even though he would stay there for almost a decade. He traveled back to Boston on weekends to see his wife and daughter, making a temporary home for himself with his Great Dane, Yonnie, who eventually bit one of the anesthesiologists. Since the lab was already packed with outraged baboons, pound dogs, and calves used in heart-related experiments, this assault was probably just one in an ongoing series of small and fruitless rebellions against the human race.

Norman brought one item of great value with him: an LVAD he had been working on with another doctor in Boston. The device had been fabricated by Thermo Electron, a company in Waltham, Massachusetts, that had been the first recipient of a federal grant to work on an artificial heart back in 1966. It wasn't a medical device company but an engineering firm focused on thermodynamics and creating nuclear power sources for space probes. They knew how to make pumps, and the heart, after all, was just another pump.

The company successfully competed against several others for NIH artificial heart grants by promoting a nuclear power source for an artificial heart—a pump driven by a miniature steam engine heated by a kernel of plutonium covered with a lead shield. Working with Norman, Thermo Electron had already reached the animal trial stage: Norman had brought a baboon who had been implanted with an experimental plutonium power source—basically, a super-battery that might eventually be applied to drive medical devices inside the human body. "Fred," as he was known to his colleagues, enjoyed watching game shows and soap operas on his black-and-white TV. Even so, he was reported to be very, very mean.

Only a certain kind of person could find paradise in this kind of workplace, and Bud Frazier was that kind. At first the lab was just a respite from the pressures of the operating room—Bud would occasionally rescue a particularly irresistible lab dog and take it home to the consternation of Rachel, or he would practice reciting Shakespearean soliloquies on a comely technician.

But the lab was also one of the few places in the world at the time where Bud could focus on his particular obsession: devices that either aided or replaced the human heart. Pretty soon he was putting the machines in lab animals and, thanks partly to Dr. Norman, working with a Thermo Electron engineer by the name of Vic Poirier, a man as self-created as Bud.

Small, intense, and bespectacled, with a thatch of brown hair and a brushy matching mustache, Poirier was hyper where Bud was laconic. He had an entrepreneur's mindset: when the shrinking space program convinced him that he was going to lose his job on a NASA project, Poirier bought himself a physiology book and a medical dictionary and talked his way into a position at Thermo Electron, as part of a team working to develop an early artificial heart. It wasn't long before Poirier became obsessed with the havoc heart disease was wreaking across the United States. It also didn't escape his notice that LVADs, which he believed might sell for around $50,000 each, could result in a market worth about $2 billion a year.

Soon enough, Poirier and Frazier became the Mutt and Jeff of heart assist devices: one didn't have the slightest grasp of engineering principles, and the other had learned about medicine from reading textbooks. But somehow, together, they started making progress. Throughout the 1970s, they inched forward, through bench testing (refining the design before animal experiments) and then by successfully implanting their device in calves, until finally they thought they had something ready to put in a person.

These trials were no longer the kind of seat-of-the-pants experiments of Bud's early days in DeBakey's lab. By the 1970s, problems with pacemakers and intrauterine devices had caused the FDA to increase regulation of medical devices, with complex machines like heart assist devices being among the most highly regulated of all.

The challenges of developing an assist device were not so different from that of a total artificial heart. The two biggest problems had never changed: a man-made pump had to have the endurance of a real heart, meaning it had to be strong enough to pump five to eleven liters of blood per minute all day, every day. Then there was the blood itself: if it wasn't moving, it was clotting, and clots that lodged in the wrong places could block circulation, and kill.

One device they came up with was designed mainly to save patients in postoperative shock following heart surgery (known as postcardiotomy shock), something that could take over the heart function while the heart itself took time to rest and recover. If that plan worked, the thinking went, maybe the same device could be used to keep patients alive while they waited for a transplant.

What they developed aped the structure of the normal heart, at least in a fashion. An air compressor that looked a little like a lectern on wheels powered the machine; a drive line extended from that console into the body via the abdomen. Attached to the left side of the heart, the inner workings of the actual device were encased in a long, narrow titanium alloy shell that looked like something more at home as part of a kitchen sink. Inside, a two-chambered pump used something called a pusher plate to draw compressed air into a chamber on one side of the device and then push it out again through the other as the air was released. This pulsing action pushed against the heart itself, literally pushing the blood through the heart and out into the aorta and the rest of the body.

Eventually Frazier, working with Cooley and Norman, implanted the LVAD in twenty-two people from 1975 through 1980. Every one of them died. Many of the patients were hopeless from the get-go; they were just too sick.

A second device worked poorly because neither Bud nor the engineers working alongside him could regulate the airflow, so the pump wore out in a few months instead of lasting the two years Bud hoped would make the device useful for a patient waiting for a transplant. Then too, the pump still wasn't powerful enough to keep the blood flowing at a consistent rate, so the danger of fatal clots loomed large.

Bud brooded on these problems constantly: when he was transplanting hearts, when he talked with Poirier, and at night when he was alone in the lab, letting the dogs out of their cages and rolling with them on the floor.

It was a less than happy memory of Dr. DeBakey that helped him solve the problem. Once during his residency, he had had to call DeBakey to see a very sick patient whose leg had grown cold after heart surgery, a sure sign his blood wasn't circulating and a blockage had formed. It was the middle of the night, and Bud was so tired that he forgot the first law of dealing with his chief: never ask DeBakey a question. Actually, he wasn't asking DeBakey, he was talking to himself, but DeBakey overheard him wondering aloud why the blood kept clotting. He whirled around and punched Bud in the chest. "Listen to me," DeBakey hissed as he kept punching. "When blood stops moving it clots. When. Blood. Stops. Moving. It. Clots. Is that too hard for your pea-sized brain?" So what was stopping the blood from moving now?

Bud looked at drawings, looked at the device, and talked with Poirier again and again. The airflow issue was improved thanks to Bud's early experience with tuberculosis patients at the Veterans Administration hospital. There, he had met a drunk who liked to frequent local bars and bet patrons he could hold his breath underwater longer than anyone else. Who could resist? Soon enough, someone brought out a bucket of water, money was collected, and two guys—the drunk and his mark—had their heads underwater. But while one man turned blue, the vet released a valve that opened a tube in his chest to the air, allowing him to breathe from this secondary location. Needless to say, he always won as long as he kept changing bars.

Maybe, Bud thought, there was a way to vent the airflow and lessen the pressure, so the pump wouldn't wear out so fast. The engineers went to work, and on the next incarnation of the LVAD, there was a tube that vented air back to the outside through the chest.

They tried the new, improved pump on patients who were waiting for, but weren't expected to live until they could get, a heart transplant. The first two died. But the third, a Miami police officer, made it. Yes, it was hard to locate his actual body what with all the tubes and wires coming in and out. And yes, the patient could not be separated from the very large operating console, which gave him the look of an oratory contest winner in a mental hospital. But he lived. Not only that, the device kept him alive and reasonably healthy until he got his new, human heart. After that, he went home. It would take more than a decade before a version of that pneumatically powered device, christened the HeartMate I, was approved as a bridge to transplantation by the Food and Drug Administration, the first time an LVAD made it across the finish line.

Bud busied himself elsewhere. In 1981, Norman had headed back to Boston without Yonnie, who preferred life with the THI janitor. There was really only one person to take over the research lab: Cooley tapped Bud to run the place. Now, when Bud wasn't transplanting hearts in the OR, he was running artificial heart research at the premier heart hospital in the world. He was forty-one. Everyone knew if you needed to get something done, Bud Frazier would do it, no matter how hard or seemingly impossible.

BARNEY WHO?

Going to an American Society for Artificial Internal Organs conference with Bud Frazier is like going to the Oscars with Jack Nich-
olson or the Super Bowl with Joe Namath: he's a celebrity, but of
the éminence grise variety. There's always a Leonardo DiCaprio or
a Tom Brady who might be younger and sexier, but even they have
to pay homage to the person who paved the way. Here, that means
frequent allusions to a phrase popularized in the seventeenth century
by Isaac Newton: "If I have seen further, it is by standing on the
shoulders of giants." It's a medical and scientific bromide, despite
equally common if less public accusations of stealing and/or refusing
to give credit where it's due.

ASAIO is the reality-based organization for the sci-fi fantasies
that have given rise to so many comic book heroes like Iron Man, as
well as the career of Lee Majors, who played the Six Million Dollar
Man in the 1970s TV hit. These are the folks who really believe that
it's only a matter of time before all of our organs can be replaced with
mechanical devices. Willem Kolff, not surprisingly, was the found-
ing president in 1955, nearly a decade after inventing the first dialysis
machine and two years before he put that artificial heart in a dog.

John Gibbon, the inventor of the first heart-lung machine, was a member too, as were Adrian Kantrowitz, who invented the balloon pump that was a precursor to the artificial heart, and Cooley. Today, members include everyone who is anyone in the world of artificial organs, which means a lot of mostly anonymous people working on everything from pacemakers to dialysis machines to heart-lung machines, from new biomaterials to artificial cells and beyond. Work on organ replacement was, like so much else, the sole purview of white men for most of the twentieth century—Bud, a past president, wears under his name tag a blue ribbon designating him as a "pioneer"—but the crowd at the San Francisco Hyatt for the 2016 conference skews young and international. There is even a smattering of women, mostly young, but including Kantrowitz's widow, Jean, a sharp, charming wonder who at ninety-two has no noticeable replacement parts. Everyone wants to talk to Bud, especially the younger folks, and they listen indulgently when he launches into one of his shaggy dog stories (Uncle Mule figures prominently), only occasionally glancing sideways at one another.

Bud is in his element, his ostrich-skin boots shined to a glistening ebony, his beloved Borsalino tipped at a rakish angle on his head. He tries to downplay his delight with all the attention—"It's like being a whore in the Klondike," he says—but also surveys the size and mix of the crowd in the plush, chandeliered ballroom with wonder. "There's hardly anybody here from the seventies," he says. "When I started out it was all the kidney people. I used to know everybody here." Sometimes he dozes through presentations, only to awaken to study a slide—"Poor goats," he says, glancing at a research presentation before returning to his nap. Other times he's like a sniper who has just put his victim in the crosshairs. Presentations that vex Bud start with a muttering monologue in his seat and then, inevitably, wind up with an extended soliloquy at the microphone during the

Q&A session. There, in his West Texas drawl, Bud proceeds to re-duce the most confident speaker to a sputtering mess. "What's your survival rate?" he demands of an inventor of children's heart pumps, sounding almost DeBakeyesque.

At least, that's how it goes until Bud runs into Robert Jarvik, with whom he has worked off and on for much of his professional life. Jarvik was born in 1946 and was probably the last medical media star after his artificial heart kept Seattle dentist Barney Clark alive for 112 days in 1982. Jarvik is six years younger than Frazier but looks a lot frailer. He is pale and wan, and has the careful walk of someone for whom a fall could be disastrous. His blue eyes are red-rimmed and a little rheumy, but his gaze remains level and piercing, especially when he is explaining his latest heart pump. These days, Jarvik may not be a household name to anyone under forty-five, but he has continued to work on the artificial heart and various assist de-vices. When Bud sidles up to his booth in the basement of the Hyatt, Jarvik brightens considerably.

The best way to explain their relationship is that they are "fren-emies." For decades, they worked together on various pumps, Jarvik refining and sending his designs to Bud at THI for testing in the lab.

Now they joke—probably incomprehensibly to anyone outside ASAIO—about, for instance, the fifty bench tests they did on a de-vice before putting it in a calf who promptly died. In another bovine joke, Jarvik suggests that Bud showcase a long-lived research calf in Houston's upcoming rodeo.

All of this is more interesting to Bud than the Barney Clark saga, the subject of which can cause him to respond with one of his ex-tended XXXL yawns. It's hard to tell whether the story bores him or exhausts him; either or both could be true. After all, Bud was there when Cooley implanted a second artificial heart in 1981, something virtually no one remembers but which, in Bud's mind, paved the way for the events in Utah. And, of course, there's this: Barney Clark's surgery has long been perceived as a screwup that set back artificial heart development for decades.

—⌇—

"The Artificial Heart Is Here," *Life* proclaimed on its cover in September 1981. The photograph showed a creepy-looking two-sided plastic device with two holes on each unit and a lot of clear plastic tubing, like something evocative of Jules Verne's *20,000 Leagues Under the Sea*. The two sides were partly held together with Velcro, which, if you thought about it, would not have been very reassuring. The cover promised "exclusive pictures of Dr. Cooley's historic heart surgery," which the magazine had been invited to see. (The second story featured on the cover asked whether women could "cut it in the military.")

As far as the general public knew at the time, the artificial heart had been in exile since Cooley had implanted the stolen heart in Haskell Karp in 1969. In the aftermath, DeBakey had put a serious hex on his future. Cooley received mild censures—but still censures—from the American College of Surgeons and the National Institutes of Health. The Harris County Medical Society issued a censure of its own, as, of course, did Baylor, which eventually led to Cooley's resignation from the faculty. Cooley rationalized the outcome of all the investigations—he insisted that his colleagues found that physicians had the right to do whatever they thought was necessary to save their patients, but many believe that Cooley's legacy as a surgeon was irrevocably damaged by his not wholly undeserved reputation as a cowboy.

It certainly hadn't helped that Mrs. Karp, once bewitched by the

Cooley charm, turned around and sued him for malpractice in 1972. She lost for a lot of reasons, but the main one was probably that the star witness for Cooley was Michael DeBakey himself, who refused to testify against his former colleague on the witness stand. As abusive as he might have been in his operating rooms and on rounds, DeBakey had no intention of questioning another doctor's decision-making in public. (The story that sounds apocryphal but actually isn't is that the plaintiff's lawyer asked Cooley to name the best heart surgeon in the world, and Cooley named himself—because, he said, he had sworn to tell the whole truth.)

But Cooley had had enough of the artificial heart business. He was quickly becoming a master of a new kind of heart surgery called the coronary bypass. The bypass was for a time almost a rite of passage for middle-aged, overstressed executives who turned up in their cardiologists' offices with blocked blood flow to their hearts and, as a result, the stabbing pain known as angina. To get the blood moving again, a surgeon builds a graft around the blocked artery, in the same way a contractor might build a new road alongside one washed out in a flood or blocked by a boulder. More than one artery can suffer a blockage, requiring a double, triple, or even quintuple bypass. By 1989, it would account for more than 60 percent of open-heart surgeries done at St. Luke's, and at a cost of around $60,000, it was certainly one of the most remunerative. As usual, Cooley could perform the procedure faster than any other doc in the United States, and he set up another assembly line that allowed him to do even more. At one time, surgeons at THI were doing thirty cases of open-heart surgery a day, mostly bypasses. In Houston, having a "Cooley tattoo" became a badge of honor, at least until statin drugs like Lipitor proved a simpler and more effective way to control the problem in the 1990s.

But Cooley never gave up on the idea of an artificial heart entirely—in fact, he never quite got over the fact that what he viewed as a medical breakthrough was seen by many of his colleagues as an unmitigated disaster and, possibly, a violation of the Hippocratic oath. The Karp implant, he wrote in an essay in 1979, "should have stimulated further clinical trials under identical conditions. Unfortunately, it seemed to deter other surgeons from being bolder in their efforts to prolong life in dying patients. . . . In some cardiac centers today, countless opportunities to gain much needed human experience are being wasted while philosophers and critics ponder the social implications." The increase in medical malpractice lawsuits "against those of us who are trying to make scientific progress" also galled him: "Regrettably, in the future many innovators in the surgical profession, as well as corporations that provide support by introducing new technologies, will be discouraged. . . . The medical profession is under extremely close scrutiny, and the demand for governmental control will, in my opinion, cause a serious handicap for future investigators."

Once again, Cooley was not going to take orders from anybody, especially the US government.

In fact, Cooley had wasted no time replacing his first replacement heart once Domingo Liotta headed back to Argentina in 1971. Cooley brought on board Tetsuzo Akutsu, a well-regarded Japanese surgeon and inventor whose work on the artificial heart dated back to 1957; it was Akutsu who worked with Kolff to implant one in a dog.

Akutsu arrived in 1974 and quickly became yet another oddball rolling through the halls of the Texas Heart Institute. He was reserved and secretive—"paranoid" was a word some used—maybe because he believed his ideas had already been pilfered under Kolff at the Cleveland Clinic. Akutsu had come to Houston via the University of Mississippi, seduced by Cooley's reputation as a surgeon as well as his willingness to try anything to keep a patient alive. Akutsu knew that if he built a working artificial heart, Denton Cooley would not let it go to waste.

At first Cooley seemed happy to wait for a flawless finished device. When he ran into Akutsu on his Saturday visits to the Texas Heart Institute, he always had the same question. "Ted," he would ask, "are you ready to put this heart in a human?" Akutsu always had the same answer: No, he was not. Unlike Cooley, Akutsu was deliberate and methodical, passionate about research, and, most of all, a perfectionist.

To Bud's way of thinking, all of these early devices were pretty much the same, partly because of the limitations of technology at the time, and partly because a certain degree of adaptation, or borrowing, of ideas was common. Akutsu's, in fact, was not substantially different from the one implanted in Karp in 1969. It was about the size of two fists, with two air-powered double-chambered pumps made of a plastic approved for medical use. A synthetic membrane filled the chambers with compressed air; one chamber pumped blood to the lungs, the other through the arteries into the rest of the body. There were special valves for inflow and outflow of the blood, and the prosthetic ventricles were attached to the actual atria and veins by flexible tubing with detachable connectors.

The device affixed to an external power console via Dacron velour tubes. The console itself had three basic parts: a pneumatic driver (an air compressor), an electrical monitoring system to measure the heart rate and heartbeat, and an electrical power system that ran on a standard electrical current with a backup battery. The console was about the size of a refrigerator, albeit one with lots of dials and gauges.

Left on his own, Akutsu continued to refine his machine, reducing the size of the control unit and the size of the heart itself, the better to fit it in a human as opposed to a calf. Within a year or so, by 1975, he had put the heart in one hundred calves and implanted it for size in the chests of twenty human cadavers, but he still wasn't satisfied. His device could never be a total replacement heart, he believed. It could, however, keep a patient alive while he or she waited for a transplant. Most of all, Akutsu worried that his heart would be tested on a human too soon. If it was, and it failed, he knew he might never be allowed to try again.

But Cooley was itchy. There is a vast divide between those who design devices and those who use them. Engineers in the medical field—actually, all engineers—want to create foolproof things, especially as the world has grown more litigious and investment capital more scarce. Doctors, on the other hand, are in a hurry—they want to save lives and work the bugs out later. Cooley, certainly, could never resist any new mechanical advance, but there were other reasons to rush. At the Cleveland Clinic, Dr. Yukihiko Nose had perfected an artificial heart that had kept a calf alive for a record-breaking seventeen days. Out at the University of Utah, a team headed by Willem Kolff was working on its own artificial heart, one designed not as a bridge to a transplant but as a permanent replacement. As the 1970s began drawing to a close, Cooley started showing up at Akutsu's office several times a week. "Is it ready?" he wanted to know.

Finally Akutsu decided it was. The finished product was sterilized. Then it sat entombed in a file cabinet, where it waited for its star turn. Cooley wasn't worried about performing preliminary animal testing. "Why should I spend time sewing it into a cow?" Cooley asked at the time. "You don't even need a medical degree for that."

Meanwhile, the headlines kept coming from the West. "Utah Doctors to Try Mechanical Heart," claimed one. "Surgeons Are Ready for Mechanical Heart Transplant," read another. Kolff's team, it was rumored, had submitted a proposal to the University of Utah's Institutional Review Board, the ethics committee that would decide whether or not the team could go forward.

Tuesday, July 21, 1981, was a typical stifling summer day in

Houston. Akutsu was making plans to move back to Japan to begin a prestigious new job when he got a frantic call from Cooley's secretary. Cooley needed him in the ICU immediately. Akutsu threw on a pair of scrubs and raced to the intensive care unit, where he found Cooley trying frantically to save a heart patient who showed every sign of dying. His pupils looked fixed, and, off and on, his EKG would go flat.

"Are you ready with that thing?" Cooley asked. "That thing" was, of course, Akutsu's mothballed heart. And Cooley wasn't really asking. Akutsu sprinted to his office; meanwhile, the surgeons rushed their patient to the operating room, tore out the stitches from his earlier surgery, and reached into his chest, trying to keep his real heart alive by massaging it rhythmically by hand.

The patient, Willebrordus Meuffels, a thirty-six-year-old Dutch tour bus driver with thick eyebrows and dark wavy hair, had been flown into Houston from the Netherlands in a special government-subsidized airlift to receive a bypass operation. Somehow it had become an article of faith among Dutch doctors that it was cheaper to fly desperately ill heart patients on a medically equipped KLM jet to Houston twice a month than to risk inferior results at home. For five years, beginning in 1976, more than fifteen hundred heart patients, mostly men aged forty-five to sixty, arrived at St. Luke's for what was at best lifesaving coronary care and at worst a marketing opportunity designed to burnish THI's reputation. Most of the patients, like Meuffels, were close to death before they even boarded their flight to Houston. It was a dark joke at THI that it was best to get them back on a plane ASAP after surgery so they could expire back home, or at least on the plane.

Meuffels' bypass surgery had seemed successful at first. Cooley sewed three pieces of vein cut from one of Meuffels' legs to replace three clogged coronary arteries. But five hours later, around two-thirty in the afternoon, he had suffered a massive heart attack. The doctors tried injecting him with drugs to restart his heart, and followed that with heart massage. But when he still did not respond, Cooley had sent Akutsu racing back to his office for his artificial heart.

One thing that Cooley did not do was seek approval from the FDA to proceed. He was well aware of new FDA restrictions on medical devices; he'd been partly to blame with the Karp implant, but problems with the intrauterine device (the IUD) had also added to stricter controls. The FDA now limited when certain devices could and could not be used, and made a clear delineation between emergency use and experimental use and the requirements for each.

Cooley could not have been less interested. He had slipped out of so many controversies by that time that his belief in asking for forgiveness instead of permission was his standard operating procedure. In his mind, waiting for bureaucratic approval could not be allowed to trump saving, or at least attempting to save, a life. As he would note a few months later, "If a man is overboard and someone throws him a life preserver, he's not going to inspect it and see if it has a guarantee."

Within an hour and a half, the Akutsu heart was pulsing successfully in Meuffels' chest, and twelve years after Haskell Karp's surgery, Denton Cooley had completed the world's second artificial heart implantation.

That was the good news. But then Cooley's team couldn't wean Meuffels off the heart-lung machine. Every time they tried, his heart stopped pumping blood to the lungs, which resulted in hypoxia, as oxygen stopped flowing to the body's tissues. Bud, assisting in surgery, jerry-rigged a temporary fix, but he and the other twenty-five medical people in the room realized that, overall, the Akutsu heart was just too big on Meuffels' body. While Meuffels remained heavily sedated, the doctors put out the word for a human heart. If he was to survive, he would need a transplant. Immediately if not sooner.

The implantation took place on Thursday; a donor heart was found on Saturday. A twenty-nine-year-old Nashville man had been left brain-dead after an auto accident. (The concept of brain death was still so novel—or frightening—after nearly two decades that the term showed up in quotes in newspaper stories of the time.) His body was flown into Houston's Hobby Airport aboard a Learjet and then helicoptered to the Texas Heart Institute. By this time, Meuffels had been alive with an artificial heart for fifty-four hours.

It took Cooley about an hour and fifteen minutes to remove it. When he was done, Akutsu held his bloody device aloft for the *Life* photographer, his expression triumphant behind his mask and glasses. During the next hour, Cooley sewed the donor heart in place. The team gathered around Meuffels, staring into the massive bloody chasm that ran the length of his chest. No one spoke.

Then, as if on cue, Meuffels' new heart began to beat, pulsing impatiently, like a child awakening from a dream too soon. Everyone who had been watching the surgery from the gallery above started clapping furiously.

But then, just as quickly, Meuffels began to fail. By the following Sunday he had a raging infection, and his kidneys and lungs were barely functioning. He was able to breathe only with the help of a respirator, and he lay in the ICU amid a thicket of tubes, wires, and IV poles. On the one hand, the surgery was miraculous: Meuffels lived significantly longer than Haskell Karp, who survived for only a day and a half after being transplanted. And Meuffels was the only man in history to have survived for a week with three different hearts, as *Life* jubilantly reported. But the prognosis wasn't good. A journalist reported that Meuffels was "barely able" to squeeze his wife's hand; in truth, he never regained consciousness. By Sunday morning, August 2, he was gone. Still, Meuffels' wife was grateful. "I have never seen so much effort for one human life," she told Cooley and his team.

They didn't know at the time how lucky they were—lucky that their patient died.

—∿—

Gratitude was not, in fact, a universal reaction. Out in Utah, the team that included Robert Jarvik and a surgeon by the name of William DeVries had been furiously working on their own artificial heart under the direction of Willem Kolff. This heart was, ostensibly, different from the one used by Cooley: it was devised for permanent use, not as a bridge to transplant. The distinction was important, because it required the Utah team to follow the strict rules set out by the FDA for permanent rather than emergency use. In other words, they weren't cowboys out in Utah. These guys played by the rules.

For the last few months, the team had been scrupulously attending to the questions posed by the Utah Medical Center's Institutional Review Board, which, in turn, would be used to make their formal request to the FDA. They all had a lot on the line: Kolff was ready to make the successful implantation of the artificial heart the crowning achievement of his career. His faith in engineering and mechanical devices—"the body as an entity of replaceable parts," in the words of medical historian Shelley McKellar—had never been shaken, despite limited success. "If a man can grow a heart, he can build one," Kolff famously stated.

The university had lured Kolff to Utah by offering him the post of chief of its new, custom-designed Institute for Biomedical Engineering and the Division of Artificial Organs. He'd been working in Utah since 1967, after a falling-out with administrators at the Cleveland Clinic over their commitment to his artificial heart research. Kolff soon showed himself to be a difficult leader, a demanding taskmaster in the DeBakey mold. He also believed in management by creative tension—pitting designers and researchers in his lab against one another. Kolff knew that government enthusiasm for the artificial heart was waning, with priorities shifting toward LVADs, and that he had to keep interest high if he wanted to keep his lab and his position. By the early 1980s, he was promising doctors and hospitals that his mechanical heart would be available soon. Very soon.

DeVries, in contrast, was a lanky, hollow-cheeked Mormon, gregarious and righteously ambitious in the mold of the heart surgeons of the day. A comer at only thirty-seven, he was already chief of cardiothoracic surgery at the University of Utah medical center. He'd worked with Kolff while in med school, then trained at Duke before returning to Kolff's exacting tutelage. DeVries had implanted artificial hearts hundreds of times in animals. Now he had a shot at making medical history, joining the pantheon of famed heart surgeons like Christiaan Barnard and Denton Cooley.

But it was Robert Jarvik, creator of this artificial heart, who had the most to prove. Few doubted his inventive genius. But he was, to put it mildly, unconventional. As Bud would frequently suggest, damning with faint praise, "Jarvik was a brilliant machinist." What he said less often but would be proven true in time was that Jarvik was not good at playing well with others—if, in fact, he played at all. He could be moody, arrogant, and/or inappropriate in his responses. He had an eerie, inopportune giggle.

At thirty-five, Jarvik also possessed an almost feminine beauty— shaggy but shimmering auburn hair, piercing blue eyes—and a restless intensity, a combination that women found irresistible. (And he them.) He had grown up watching his father perform surgery and, like Cooley, had been an inveterate tinkerer. (His uncle, Murray Jarvik, was an inventor of the nicotine patch.) By the time Jarvik graduated from high school, he had already invented an automatic stapler to replace suturing in surgery. While at Syracuse University in 1964,

Jarvik considered a career in architecture, and also showed gifts as a sculptor and designer. Then his father developed heart disease, and he switched to medicine.

Gifted though he was, Jarvik had issues, predominantly with rules and structure, which prevented him from finishing med school, even the one in Bologna he was enrolled in after he couldn't get admitted to any American school. ("I am a medical scientist, not a practical physician," he declared at one point, a statement few colleagues would dispute.) He finally ended up with a master's degree in biomechanics from New York University, when Kolff found him and brought him to Utah as a designer in his lab; it was with Kolff's help that Jarvik finally obtained a medical degree from the University of Utah in 1976. He never completed an internship or residency; instead, he joined Kolff's artificial organ team full-time.

On Thursday, July 23, 1981, as he was enjoying an evening with friends, Robert Jarvik's future looked as bright and shining as the desert sky outside Salt Lake, where he made his home. Then his phone rang. It was William DeVries, who had just gotten a call from a reporter. Denton Cooley had implanted an artificial heart in a patient in Houston. The reporter wondered whether DeVries would care to comment. Now DeVries waited for Jarvik's response.

"Well, that is one of the most interesting things I've heard in ages," Jarvik said in a voice as dry as the desert air.

Kolff, who knew Cooley well and had supported putting the heart in Haskell Karp, was more gracious. "Congratulations," he telegraphed Cooley, and with Old World panache added, "Well done. Save the patient's life while you are blazing the trail. Best wishes for your patient, my fellow Dutchman, and for you from all of us in Utah."

DeVries had a similar reaction. "It would take someone like Cooley to stand up to the review board and the FDA," he said. In fact, Cooley had gotten around the FDA by declaring the surgery experimental, despite the fact that he had been hounding Akutsu to finish his device for years. But that independence—or insubordination, depending on your point of view—would prove to be the silver lining for the Utah team, at least initially. Cooley's end run might help them speed up their own approval process, which by then had been dragging on for a couple of years. It stood to reason that with two other "experimental" implants completed, the Utah device looked less radical, more reasonable, more considered, and more responsible.

Like most inventors, Jarvik drew on the past for his design. He cast his net so widely, in fact, that some of his work came from an artificial heart created by Paul Winchell, whose reputation as an inventor was eclipsed by his talent as a ventriloquist—his partner in the 1950s was dummy Jerry Mahoney. At Kolff's direction, Jarvik also drew on the work of Dr. Clifford Kwan-Gett, who was a member of the Utah team and had worked with Kolff previously on a design for an artificial heart.

The first three hearts Jarvik designed never reached the animal testing stage. A fourth, called the pancake heart, had flatter sides than the Liotta or Akutsu heart but, like these hearts (and the Kwan-Gett heart, for that matter), worked with air pumped into the device through plastic tubes from an external compressor. Inside, razor-thin rubber membranes sat atop one another, forming a diaphragm that opened and closed with the force of the air. A graphite lubricant was used to keep the surface flexible; another substance was used to prevent life-threatening clots.

The first hearts Jarvik made with this design were too big for humans; they were designed to operate in calves. Eventually he made a smaller heart that came to be known as the Jarvik-7. (Kolff liked to name his devices after students and assistants who worked on them, a tribute that would come to rank high in the No Good Deed Goes Unpunished chronicles.)

All told, the Kolff team completed more than 360 animal experiments. Over time, the life span of the calves (and a sheep or two) extended from a few weeks to several months. A calf named Abebe lived for six months in 1977. One named Alfred Lord Tennyson lived nearly nine.

The most obvious problem with the Jarvik-7—though others would be discovered later—was the air compressor. This heart was a shotgun marriage of man and machine: a patient would be tethered to a device the size of a dishwasher for the rest of his or her life. This was, after all, supposed to be a *permanent* artificial heart. Like most compressors, it also made a lot of noise, constantly. This didn't bother Kolff, who pointed out that there were thousands of paraplegics and quadriplegics in the United States who had adapted to much worse.

But this aspect had bothered the university's Institutional Review Board, the ethics committee charged with supervising any human testing and that first step in winning FDA approval. Under the tightened FDA rules formulated in the 1980s, the Jarvik-7 was classified as an investigational device, which meant its use posed "a potential for serious risk to the health, safety, or welfare of a patient" and was of "unproven safety and efficacy." In a classic example of words coming back to haunt the author, Jarvik himself had written an article for *Scientific American* in January 1981 stating that no artificial heart, including those he was still working on, was ready for human implantation. The review board raised lots of other questions too, about many of the problems that had plagued experimental artificial hearts all along: the incompatibility of various biomaterials, the durability of various parts, the frequency of infection, and, yes, that pneumatic console. Further, the board wasn't impressed with the life span of the calves with Jarvik-7s: they preferred a life span of two years instead of nine months. (Future regulators would rescind such a requirement once longer survival rates showed that calves outgrew their artificial hearts in about ninety days.)

While they waited, the team tested the fit in human cadavers, and even tested it in brain-dead patients.

In addressing the doubts of the review board, the Kolff team posited that some of the problems might be more common to calves than humans, and that the infection rates probably came from bacteria in the animal lab. More to the point, federal funds for artificial heart creation were running out or being shifted elsewhere. Time was running out. They had to move.

After many revisions over the next six months, the review board finally gave consent to proceed in February 1981. The FDA gave tentative approval the following fall. But then no patients could be found who matched their stringent criteria. This person had to be nearly—but not completely—dead from heart disease. It was a requirement that would plague many human trials: who could tell if an operation failed because the patient was too weak to survive surgery, or because a device just didn't work? In June 1982, the FDA loosened the rules, but still attached some pretty serious strings: the patient had to be terminally ill with congestive heart failure and unsuitable for a transplant. In other words, have no choice but to try a machine for a heart.

There were some dissenting voices among cardiac surgeons about the wisdom of moving ahead. Cooley was one of them. It must have galled the Utah surgeons that as they were finally closing in on government approval, Cooley wrote an article for *American Medical News*, claiming that "the artificial heart is not ready for elective implantation and cannot even approach the expectation of cardiac transplantation today." He had a point: with the success of the immunosuppressant cyclosporin A, more and more transplant patients were making it with their new hearts. A Palo Alto group was reporting a 70 percent survival rate.

The delays in implanting the Jarvik-7 continued. In something of a reverse beauty contest, it took seven months to find an appropriate volunteer, even with the softened restrictions. As a headline in *People* put it, "Utah Surgeon William DeVries Seeks a Patient Who Could Live with a Man-Made Heart." Psychiatrists were brought in to examine the prospects, along with other medical personnel; the team of evaluators determined that the perfect patient should have the risk-taking, adventure-seeking "right stuff"—the term popularized in Tom Wolfe's 1979 book about NASA's test pilots and the first astronauts. They actually used some of NASA's screening procedures for astronauts to look for the right heart patient.

It was as if they were trying to cast a Hollywood film about American grit in the face of adversity, and maybe they were: during the search for the ideal candidate, the PR department of the University of Utah started gearing up for the significant attention they assumed would come in the wake of the surgery. They too took some cues from the NASA playbook, including the decision to provide 24/7 availability to reporters. And why not? The implantation of an artificial heart would be at least as important to humankind as a trip to the moon.

Finally they found their man: Barney Clark, a sixty-one-year-old Seattle dentist for whom the phrase "salt of the earth" seemed to have been invented. He was a tall, solid-looking fellow with a broad, open face, soft blue eyes, and a pugilist's nose. Until he developed heart disease, Clark had been a successful dentist and an avid golfer. He was self-made: he had grown up in rural Utah, and the family's modest income crashed precipitously after Clark's father, a traveling salesman, committed suicide. As a result, Clark and his mother became extremely close; he started helping with finances at the age of eleven, and grew up determined to make her proud.

The evaluators saw it as a plus that Clark had flown combat missions in World War II and had received two Bronze Stars. He had worked hard to put himself through dental school, and then worked even harder to build his practice. He had a loving wife, Una Loy, who resembled her husband in her nearly boundless optimism. They had three devoted, well-adjusted children.

Clark was, in short, a brave, thoughtful man who worked hard and wanted very much to please. In one interview, he worried "about making a fool of either myself or the university project." Before signing an eleven-page consent form, he grinned at the doctors present and said, "There sure would be a lot of long faces around here if I backed out now." He understood that he was agreeing to become a human guinea pig, and hoped that his agreement to participate would serve humanity down the road.

But, of course, he was also dying. He was too sick to walk across a room or lift an arm to brush his teeth. He had severe tachycardia—a rapid heartbeat that prevents the proper flow of blood to the rest of his body. His heart was only pumping one liter per minute, with 5–7 being the norm. A transplant wasn't an option: Clark was too old, according to medical criteria at the time. He was out of choices, except for one wildly improbable alternative. No one will ever know what Clark wished for more: to be of service in his last days, or simply to extend them regardless of the price.

DeVries implanted the Jarvik-7 on the night of December 2, 1982, under the gaze of just about the entire world. Despite the university's planning, its PR department was totally unprepared for the onslaught of print and television reporters, who came like thundering hordes, expecting yet another triumphant American success story.

Clark did well in the first twenty-four hours following surgery. His color returned, and he happily recognized visitors. Una Loy was deeply relieved: "I kept telling him how much I loved him and how happy I was he was still with us," she told the press. "I said, 'I'm so thankful. I thought because you have an artificial heart you might not still love us.'"

But by the next day doctors discovered some emphysema. Somehow, despite all its research, the evaluation committee appointed to select the first patient to receive a Jarvik-7 had failed to catch Clark's chronic obstructive pulmonary disease—a condition that was on their list of disqualifying illnesses. Now Clark's condition required a short trip back into surgery. At first he recovered nicely, and was even taken off the critical list. His dental experience came in handy as he joked with the nurses about their inability to correctly brush his teeth. He offered to buy them a round of Cokes.

After six days, however, Clark began having seizures and soon became semicomatose. Then one of the artificial mitral valves fractured, and he was rushed back into surgery. Again, Clark seemed to recover. But now, in addition to the noise of the artificial heart compressor, which emanated a constant *click-whoosh-click-whoosh*, Clark had to communicate with a tube in his throat and a respirator over his mouth. Still, he remained for the most part alert and cheerful, the hospital darling.

Over the next three weeks, though, Clark became increasingly disoriented and delusional, or displayed what the psychiatrists observing him described as a "flat affect." Then he got better—he was able to walk with a rickety gait, and even use an exercise bicycle. Una Loy would report a "joyful" Christmas with the family. But soon after, Clark became so despondent that he asked to be allowed to die. Then he became lucid again, with no memory of his request. The psychiatrists noted that "even during periods of significant despair, the patient remained cooperative, compliant, and attempted to render any self help within his capability."

By eight weeks, Clark had had three more surgical procedures and was diagnosed with "significant organic brain syndrome," which meant that he was suffering from dementia caused by a medical instead of mental disease. He was also suffering from, among other things, renal failure, pneumonia, gout, painfully swollen testicles, and an ulcer. "There is continued diminution of interest in his surroundings," the psychiatrists wrote. Clark put his situation succinctly: he felt he had "no life to live." Una Loy felt she was losing him. It was as if her husband had put up a wall between them, one she could not breach with her love.

And then, as he had in the past, Clark rallied. The light never returned to his eyes, but he could clearly describe feeling, as his wife had sensed, that he was being closed in by impenetrable walls. At other moments Clark imagined himself walking out of his hospital room, and even outside. At his most lucid, he worried about becoming a burden to his wife when he went home, and he worried about his growing hospital bill, which would eventually hit $250,000—about $700,000 today. As Una Loy wrote, "The days pass and we are still trying to climb a big hill."

In truth, no one really knew how or what Clark was feeling. Because of the brain damage, the respirator, and the tangle of tubes and wires snaking in and out of his body, he had no way to effectively communicate. Even when suffering from sepsis, renal failure, pneumonia, and gastroenteritis, he was true to his nature, keeping up a good front. "I'm still trying," he struggled to tell visitors.

Death finally came the night of March 24, 1983, as a light snow fell, visible through the windows of the surgical intensive care unit where his nurses could be seen openly weeping. He had lived 112 days with the Jarvik-7 in his chest.

Clark's funeral was a national event, with fifteen hundred people attending. Kolff gave a eulogy. Someday, he said, as many as fifty thousand Americans a year might live with artificial hearts, and "their borrowed days, weeks and years will be a precious gift from

Barney Clark and Una Loy. He taught us that the artificial heart does not hurt, that its noise is manageable. Most of all, he taught us that it did not destroy his spirit and his ability to love."

An autopsy showed that the device had worked well. The Utah team believed they had a winner.

—⋀⋀—

Their victory, however, was short-lived. Thanks to the aggressive PR efforts of the university, and probably its inexperience with the new phenomenon of media circuses, the entire world had either seen video of or read about every detail of Clark's surgery—as well as the minute details of his agonizing decline. So what was supposed to be a PR and fundraising boon turned into a massive PR disaster.

Initially, the Clark narrative was that of a medical miracle with lots of good guys, including the "Lincolnesque" surgeon DeVries, the hot, motorcycle-jacketed Jarvik, and Clark himself, who was cast as the "avuncular astronaut." (Hadn't Ed White been tethered to the mother ship when he became the first American to walk in space in 1965? Hadn't Neil Armstrong been tethered to a portable life support unit when he took his first step on the moon in 1969?) Though Clark and his family were largely shielded from the media—save for the reporter who snuck into the hospital in a laundry basket—the hospital hosted twice-daily press conferences in the basement to keep journalists and their audiences abreast of virtually every breath Clark took. News bulletins interrupted regularly scheduled programs. Jarvik and DeVries were, of course, magazine cover boys.

As the months dragged on and Clark deteriorated, the university tried to pull back on the media front. It was too late. Barney Clark's story became one of dashed hope as it became painfully clear that

American know-how couldn't do for the human body what it had done for space exploration. It didn't help that Clark's surgery took place in the post-Watergate era. Bob Woodward and Carl Bernstein had brought down a president with their reporting on the Watergate scandal in 1972, and now a new generation of hungry investigative reporters was focused on Utah.

At the same time, the new field of bioethics was expanding, largely because of the ever-growing intersection of technology and medicine. Congress had passed the National Research Act in 1974 in response to some highly unethical experiments on humans, in particular the infamous Tuskegee, Alabama, syphilis experiment of 1932–1972, in which 408 impoverished black men with syphilis were never treated, only observed, as they died. Part of the act included the creation of Institutional Review Boards, like the one in Salt Lake City, which were supposed to protect patients who agreed to be involved in scientific research. Now physicians weren't the only ones with the power to make life-and-death decisions. Their authority would be questioned even further with the establishment of the President's Commission for the Study of Ethical Problems in Medicine and Biomedical and Behavioral Research, issued just before Clark's surgery.

Not coincidentally, the commercialization of medical care was also a big issue at the time. Everything from the exceedingly generous public contributions to help defray the Clark family's medical bills to the University of Utah's use of PR as a fundraising tool for more implantations came under the microscope, as did the exclusive rights given to the German magazine *Stern* for the Clark story, for which the magazine paid $100,000. ("The astronauts sold their story for $500,000 to *Life* magazine," one hospital official groused.)

Then there were the problems with Kolff Medical. It was not widely known that in 1976 Kolff, Jarvik, and several associates had formed an independent company to market their artificial heart and its accompanying compressor. In fact, Jarvik had become so adept at raising millions in venture capital that he ended up in charge, elbowing Kolff out of the way and renaming the company Symbion. DeVries and the university were also stockholders, which raised significant conflict-of-interest issues.

The Institutional Review Board came under scrutiny too, as reporters uncovered more information about its decision-making process, particularly the disagreements between the doctors and the engineers over the readiness of the Jarvik heart. That eleven-page consent form presented to the Clarks was dismissed by one prominent ethicist as ridiculous. A University of Alabama ethicist called it "fishy." Was the Utah team trying to heal the sick, or was it just trying to continue a medical experiment of dubious value? Two major American sociologists, Judith P. Swazey and Renee C. Fox, conducted an independent investigation of the affair; in a book based on their research, *Spare Parts*, they wrote that putting the artificial heart in Barney Clark had been "fundamentally unethical" and "profoundly disquieting," characterized by "dangerous excesses" and "misconduct."

Things got so bad that a major symposium was held in 1984 to examine in excruciating detail the legal, ethical, medical, commercial, and journalistic sins that resulted from Clark's surgery.

But it was Barton J. Bernstein, the prominent Stanford historian, who was probably the most damning, declaring that "instead of being allowed to die peacefully," Clark "had undergone a series of painful procedures in full view of the public." More important, "there was no evidence that the massive federal investment in artificial hearts would ever truly improve the quality of life of patients."

Under cover of night, DeVries and his family moved to Louisville in 1984, where he joined the staff of a Humana hospital. The University of Utah was rethinking its commitment to the artificial heart program, and like Cooley before him, DeVries had been getting death threats. "Artificial Heart Surgeon William DeVries Transplants Himself to Greener Pastures," was the way *People* magazine described the move.

DeVries put it differently, saying that he was tired of watching "people die while I wait for the red tape." He would never waver in his belief that any kind of life was preferable to death, but it was becoming increasingly difficult to convince the federal government, and the public, that he was right.

THE PRISONER

By the 1980s, Bud had made a name for himself as both a tireless transplant surgeon and a relentless researcher. A colleague from the University of Texas had recommended him for appointment to a National Heart, Lung, and Blood Institute (NHLBI) advisory committee with the incoming Reagan administration, which, thanks largely to the Barney Clark debacle, was fast losing interest in funding total artificial hearts. A government study released in May 1982—prior to Clark's surgery—showed that Cooley's implantations had also had an influence, as had the reports from ethicists who had criticized those surgeries. There was mention of technical difficulties being greater than anticipated. No one seemed to know how to design and produce certain crucial components. There were still problems with blood destruction and the power source. "Estimates as to when a totally implantable artificial heart system capable of long term support will be achieved are uncertain. The most common forecast is 'many years away'," the study concluded. Then came the death watch for Clark.

In 1985, the director of the NHLBI canceled all federal funding for artificial heart research in favor of work on LVADs. After all, wasn't half an artificial heart better than none at all?

Over time, with more experiments and more testing, Bud and Vic Poirier began developing an LVAD that was portable—meaning a person could actually leave the hospital without dragging around an enormous console. They wanted the device to be electrically powered instead of air powered, and its outer workings small enough to be stored in something about the size of a backpack. Given the state of the technology at the time, success seemed unlikely, but by 1991 they thought they had something that worked, and Bud also had a patient willing to give it a go.

Mike Templeton was a very young but very sick man. He was thirty-two years old, from the north Houston exurb of Humble, and by the time he got to the Texas Heart Institute, he had only two choices: gamble with an experimental device or let death take him within the next day or two.

Like so many people with heart disease, Mike's problems developed very slowly and then accelerated with an almost frightening speed. Just two years or so before, he had been a strapping young man, a high school graduate who stood six feet tall and weighed 200 pounds, most of it muscle put on while he worked as a pipeline technician in the oil fields. He wore his straight brown hair brushed off his broad, open face, and aviator-style eyeglasses. His brushy mustache slipped down over the edges of his lips, suggesting a perpetual frown, but something gentle behind his eyes mitigated even a hint of disapproval or disdain. By nature, Mike was a happy-go-lucky guy who didn't want for much. He desperately loved his feisty wife, Tara, and his two daughters, Shana and Jenna.

One day he got a cold that wouldn't go away. At night, he tossed and turned with watery congestion in his chest. When he started coughing up blood, Tara demanded he see a doctor.

That's when he got the bad news. Mike had something called idiopathic cardiomyopathy; his heart muscle had become enlarged and thickened, and it was no longer strong enough to pump blood through his body. The cause was unknown. The doctors told him he needed a transplant immediately.

He stayed in the local hospital for three weeks and convinced himself that he would be all right with medication. He went home and managed to work a little, but the deterioration continued over the next few months. He was bloated, nauseated, and, again, coughing up blood. That time, Mike got as far as the hospital steps before he blacked out; the next thing he knew, he woke up in another place, St. Luke's. Doctors at the Texas Heart Institute got him stabilized and put him on the transplant list. He went home to wait.

After another near-fatal collapse—by then Mike's liver and kidneys were failing too—he was rushed back to St. Luke's via emergency helicopter. There he met Bud Frazier, who provided him with one more option: the new LVAD they had been working on in the lab. Bud was honest: they had tried the device once before, and the patient had died.

Mike was almost too weak to sign the consent form. "There must have been sixty pairs of eyes looking at me," he told *Houston Chronicle* reporter Claudia Feldman. "It was quite a day. The staff told me they were going to film the operation. They said they weren't going to let me die—I was going to be on TV."

When he woke up, Mike felt better than he had in years. He sat up the next day, and walked a few paces down the hall, the power pack slung over his shoulder, the *sss-boom, sss-boom* of the machine pulsing just above a whisper. He was stunned to the point of tears when he discovered soon after that that he could play basketball, and beat his brother Richard in a footrace.

The only downside was that Mike did both those things inside the confines of St. Luke's. The FDA had added another stipulation when it had approved emergency implantation of the new HeartMate: the device was approved as a one-time-only bridge to transplantation. Mike would not be allowed to leave the hospital until a donor heart was beating in his chest. As Frazier knew, this could take a long time: his patient was a large man, and his blood type, O positive, was the most common, which meant that the wait time for a donor heart would be the longest. (Hearts from donors with type O blood can also go to recipients with other blood types.) In the meantime, the US government required that Templeton be kept safe with an approved escort every time he left the hospital floor. Leaving the hospital itself was out of the question. Who knew if or when the pump would give out?

For a while, the rules didn't matter. Mike became something of a celebrity, since news of his surgery was reported worldwide. Strangers asked to be photographed with him in the St. Luke's lobby. Doctors asked how he was feeling. And he was so grateful to see his family. Mike seemed to have his life back, or at least he believed that he would soon. But as money grew tight without his income, he and Tara began to fight more. And as time passed, his growing girls grew less and less willing to spend their free time at the hospital. He was like an astronaut walking in space, tethered to the lifesaving mother ship but cut off from all he knew. At times he thought about making a break for it—just walking out of the hospital and taking his chances. But he realized that would leave Bud in a bind, and he couldn't do that to the man who had saved his life. Mike thought too about all the people whose lives could be saved with the device keeping him alive. He couldn't let them down either.

In fact, Frazier, Poirier, and even Cooley were furiously lobbying the FDA to release Templeton from bondage. But the answer was always no. The doctors could see Templeton was mentally deteriorating. As his time in the hospital closed in on a year, the light in his eyes faded, he shuffled, and he spoke in a monotone. His anxiety kept him awake at night, and he began to haunt the floor in the dim twilight of the hallway. He looked, in short, like a man who had stopped caring whether he lived or died. The option of a transplant terrified Templeton as well; he didn't think he could endure another medical procedure, especially as he watched many other patients leave the hospital and then come back sicker than before. And he hated the idea that someone else had to die so that he could live. "I didn't bargain for all this," he told the *Chronicle*. "But I want to see my girls grow up."

Finally, in September 1992, the FDA relented and Mike Templeton was free to go back home to Humble. He had spent more than a year in the hospital and would be remembered in the medical literature as the first patient in history to leave the hospital with a portable HeartMate I. He was alive and untethered.

But leaving the hospital is not the same as going home. The life Templeton remembered and so desperately craved to return to was gone. He had been a strong man who cared deeply about providing for his family; now they were providing for him, and the emotional and financial drain seemed, to him, insurmountable. Four months later, he stopped taking the medication that kept his blood from clotting. Almost immediately, he suffered a fatal stroke.

"The pump worked fine," Bud told the press. But Templeton's heart was completely broken.

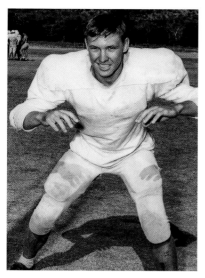

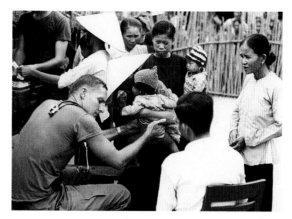

Frazier was a flight surgeon in Vietnam from 1968 to 1969 but spent his free time treating local villagers. *(Courtesy of Texas Heart Institute)*

Bud Frazier as a high school football star in West Texas, 1950s. *(Courtesy of Dr. Frazier)*

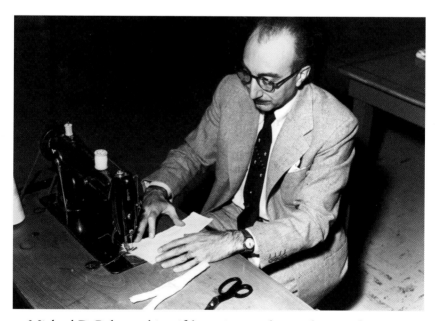

Michael DeBakey at his wife's sewing machine, where in the 1950s he created a revolutionary vascular graft. This photo was staged for posterity. *(Courtesy of Baylor College of Medicine Archives)*

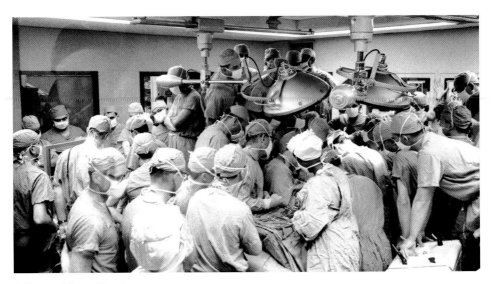

A Texas Heart Institute operating room in the 1960s. At the time, THI performed more heart surgeries than any place in the world. *(Courtesy of Texas Heart Institute)*

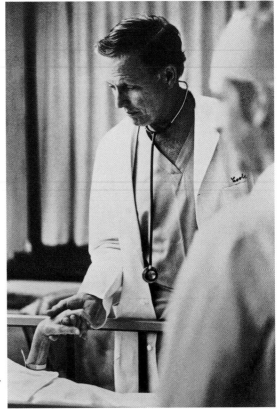

Denton Cooley bedside in the 1970s. *(Courtesy of Texas Heart Institute)*

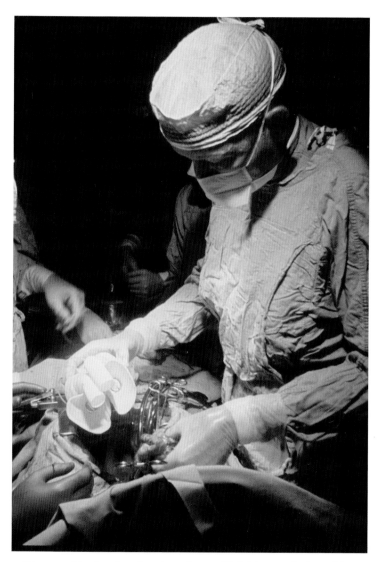

Denton Cooley implanting the artificial heart designed by
Domingo Liotta, 1969. *(Courtesy of Texas Heart Institute)*

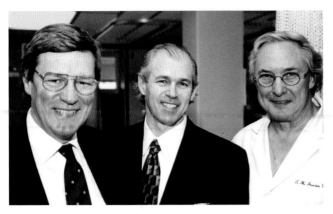

Bud Frazier with noted British heart surgeon Dr. Stephen Westaby (far left) and Dr. Robert Jarvik, inventor of the artificial heart implanted in Barney Clark in 1982. *(Courtesy of Dr. Frazier)*

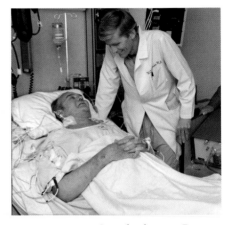

Seattle dentist Barney Clark lived for 112 days with the Jarvik-7 artificial heart. He is pictured here with his surgeon, William DeVries. *(Courtesy of Spencer S. Eccles Health Sciences Library, University of Utah)*

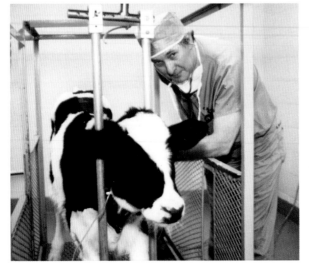

Calves have been used in the majority of artificial heart experiments because their biology is the closest to that of humans. *(Courtesy of Dr. Frazier)*

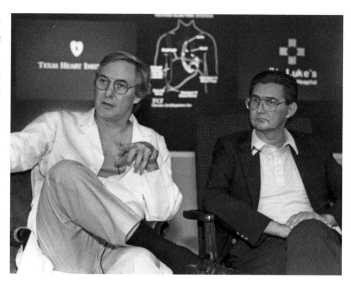

Bud Frazier with patient Mike Templeton, 1991. Templeton was the first patient to leave the hospital with a left ventricular assist device, the modern version of which has been implanted in 40,000 people. *(Courtesy of Texas Heart Institute)*

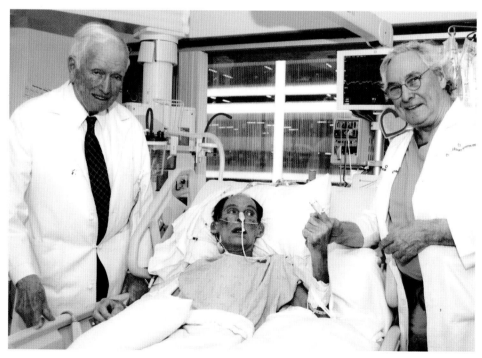

Drs. Frazier and Cooley with Craig Lewis, who lived for five weeks with two HeartMate II's put together. *(Courtesy of Dr. Frazier)*

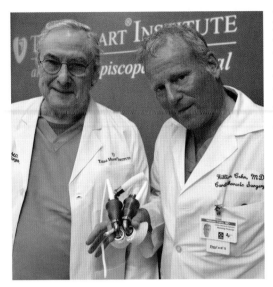

Bud Frazier and
Billy Cohn with their
total artificial heart
made by combining
two HeartMate II left
ventricular assist
devices, circa 2011.
*(Courtesy of Texas
Heart Institute)*

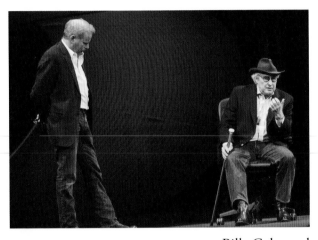

Billy Cohn and
Bud Frazier
describing their
work on artificial
hearts at TEDMED
conference, 2012.
*(Courtesy of Texas
Heart Institute)*

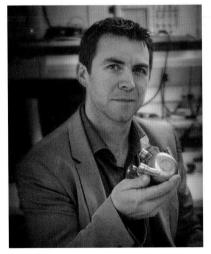

Australian biomedical
engineer Daniel Timms
holding the Bivacor,
2016. *(Courtesy of
BIVACOR Inc./Texas
Heart Institute)*

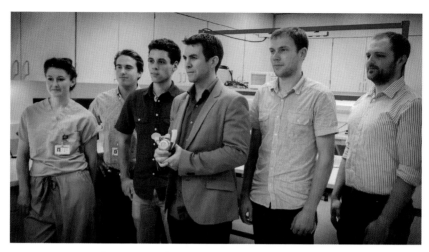

A portion of Timms' global Bivacor team in the THI lab, 2016.
(Courtesy of BIVACOR Inc./Texas Heart Institute)

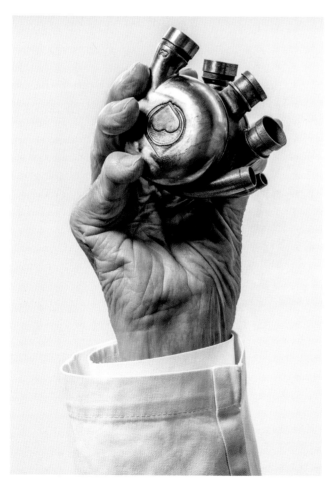

Bud Frazier's hand holding what could be the culmination of his lifelong dream, an artificial heart that might one day be mass produced to save tens of thousands of lives. *(Courtesy of Texas Heart Institute)*

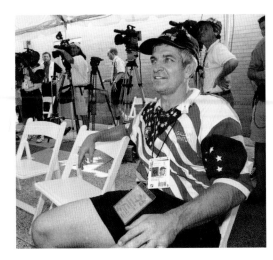

Mattress Mack, aka Jim McIngvale, in the 1980s. The furniture store mogul and philanthropist is an investor in the Bivacor. *(Associated Press)*

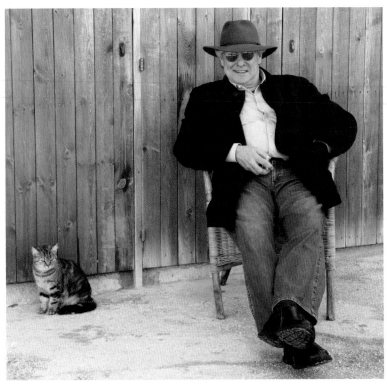

Bud Frazier in repose in West Texas, 2016.
(Courtesy of Marianne Mallia)

THE WILDERNESS

In retrospect, there were several interesting and important developments that emerged from the Templeton case. Yes, in 1994, the FDA approved pneumatically driven devices like the HeartMate I for use as a bridge to transplantation. But the most interesting and important thing might have been that Bud decided that a machine that kept a person alive by mimicking the pumping action of the natural heart wasn't the best idea for an artificial heart—even if the Heart-Mate's latest iteration was good enough to allow a patient to play tennis. That was typical of Bud, but just about everyone else in the medical community thought his alternative was crazy.

So was his timing. Since the late 1980s, the public and politicians had been trying to wash their hands of the whole idea of a totally implantable artificial heart. Everyone from members of the Reagan administration to prominent academic bioethicists was losing faith. There were several reasons for this. First, society at large didn't seem as enthralled with the miracles of the medical profession anymore; the Barney Clark media pile-on had certainly given that viewpoint a boost. So too did the so-called Baby Fae case, in which a doctor successfully transplanted a baboon heart into a human infant who lived for two weeks in 1984, setting off another ethical furor. Much closer to home but no less controversial was the death of the "Bubble Boy," David Vetter, that same year; he was more or less incarcerated with a rare autoimmune disease in a Texas Medical Center hospital from his birth in 1971 until he died at the age of thirteen. Were doctors trying to heal the sick or just experimenting on defenseless people for the most narcissistic of reasons? Or, maybe, both?

Then there was the issue of cost. The deep recession of 1980–82 was followed by deep cuts in social spending and general belt tightening for everyone. Stanford historian Bernstein took up the charge again. "Can America afford to develop a workable artificial heart?" he asked in an article in *The Nation*, suggesting that the cost of serving the "16,000–66,000 potential recipients"—a pretty broad spectrum—would range from $1.6 billion to $6.6 billion at a time when the federal deficit was approaching $200 billion. And given the ongoing but less than successful experiments with the Jarvik heart—the misery played out in public with five more patients over the next few years—people began to wonder how much better life with an artificial heart was than simply living out whatever time they had left with the faulty heart they'd been born with.

Then too, enough had been learned about heart disease by that time to suggest that preventive medicine—Stop smoking! Start jogging! Eat less meat, more vegetables!—was a much better option than heroic, Hail Mary measures once a crisis set in. Bernstein noted in his article that the artificial heart "represents a triumph of skilled physicians and technology over illness and nature. But such triumphs can be costly and shortsighted."

On the other hand, people continued to die in record numbers from heart disease. And the number of available hearts for transplants remained stuck at twenty-five hundred per year, while tens of thousands waited in desperation for a rescue that wasn't coming. These were the facts that troubled Bud a lot more than the cost of implants or the bioethicists who thought he was in league with Dr. Frankenstein.

Bud believed his patients needed something new; he just wasn't sure what that would be. All he knew was that he was ready to abandon air-powered pumps, not just for LVADs but for any future total artificial hearts he might devise. Yes, air-powered pumps paid the bills in his lab, and could keep a patient alive for a few years. But once the machine started to falter, those patients would wind up either back in surgery for replacement parts or back on the transplant list; so far, no air-powered device could equal the natural heart's ability to beat 115,000 times a day.

In addition, the current pumps were too big. No one had come anywhere close to inventing a device that could fit inside a woman's chest, much less that of a child. To Bud, the answer seemed obvious: someone had to come up with something different. A machine that kept the blood flowing through the body but didn't have a pump that wore out. Something that would flow continuously, without a break, for who knew how long. Maybe longer than the life of the patient it was implanted in.

Bud began talking about the issue with friends and colleagues, but also in public, at medical conferences, and in papers he wrote for medical journals. There were researchers and engineers who were abandoning air-powered pumps for centrifugal pumps, which forced blood through the body with a spinning instead of a pulsing action. But spinning blood at high speeds was well known to create one dangerous side effect, a condition known as hemolysis, in which red blood cells fall apart, leading to anemia and then more serious problems, like kidney and heart failure. Once again, blood destruction was looking like a barrier to success.

Another side effect of a centrifugal device would be that the patient wouldn't have a pulse, something no human being had done without since emerging from the primordial ooze. Bud's attitude was, so what? Who said you really needed it?

The answer was: the entire medical profession. Or, at least, that segment of the medical profession that studied such things, which included many of Bud's esteemed colleagues. They had tolerated all of his mumbling and grumbling, the rotating library of Penguin classics in his coat pocket, and the *Boys' Life* stories about his childhood in West Texas because Bud was a world-class surgeon. He was the one you wanted in the OR, whether you were transplanting, implanting, or just trying to keep some unlucky soul from dying in your very hands. But now, it seemed, Bud's colorful imagination had gotten the better of him. Now he was going on and on with all this pulsatile-versus-nonpulsatile nonsense. It was ridiculous. No self-respecting surgeon was going to waste time on a scheme that probably ensured his or her signature on a patient's death certificate.

What followed was a personal trial for Bud. Now forty-eight, he was keeping pace with Cooley to maintain the Heart Institute's backbreaking surgical schedule. And it was Bud, not Cooley, who was running the ever-expanding research lab down in the basement.

He had worked tirelessly to get himself to the pinnacle of his profession. The perks weren't what they had been in DeBakey's or Cooley's heyday—even in those pre-Kardashian days, magazine editors were rapidly losing interest in putting doctors on their covers unless, like the bearded, avuncular, Harvard-trained Andrew Weil, they were sporting some new, natural, organic, life-extending cure for who knew what. Still, Bud was doing pretty well: he traveled around the world, sometimes with Cooley and sometimes without, performing surgery and lecturing on the latest techniques. He knew the best restaurants in Paris, Riyadh, and God knows where else, and he had a whole entourage of minders who allowed him to focus exclusively on saving lives. The best medical journals clamored for his papers. He lived just a few blocks from Denton Cooley in a more modest but elegantly appointed home in River Oaks, and his son and daughter went to the best private school in Houston. As with so many doctors of this time, home life was something Bud mostly did without. There is a story that Rachel Frazier tells about this period that is illustrative: for some unfathomable reason, Bud had to make a run to his home in the middle of the day. Colleagues at THI would have been surprised that he found the place at all, but he managed to unlock the front door with his key and headed upstairs. There he ran into the family maid of many years, who took one look at the shambling, shaggy-haired intruder and screamed in terror. She had never seen Bud before. Still, to most small-town Texas boys—and a lot of big-city Texas boys—Dr. Bud Frazier looked like he had it made.

Until he boarded that pulseless heart train. Then, as Bud put it to a writer for *Popular Mechanics* many years later, "I was like Robinson Crusoe doing magic tricks for the goats." The man who had once won virtually all medical debates using the latest scientific data suddenly found himself trying to score points with—a feeling in his gut. This was not a good spot for a man of medicine. Oh, he argued that all the other organs operated with continuous flow; that was one point. And blood flowed continuously at the capillary level—it didn't need a pulse to keep moving there. But that was all he had. He just believed you could make a heart with continuous flow instead of a pulse. Bud had no scientific proof that humans could do without a pulse or a heartbeat, while the opposition had the entirety of medical history on its side.

Bud had a slight proclivity for aggrievement, and now he could be seen and heard complaining extensively around the Texas Heart Institute about the lack of support for his idea among his peers. He was like a very large, wounded animal. Maybe a woolly mammoth. There were people who fled when they saw Bud coming down the hall, even if he appeared to be engrossed yet again in that dog-eared copy of *Hamlet*. Bud simply could not believe that his colleagues had turned on him. He wrote more papers on continuous flow. They were summarily rejected.

It just didn't do to slack off when a breakthrough was on the horizon, even if Bud was one of the few people who realized it. Serving on the National Heart, Lung, and Blood Institute's prestigious advisory board was a help. The NHLBI was the third-largest institute within the National Institutes of Health. Soon enough, Bud found himself sitting next to Michael DeBakey, who had not spoken to him in eleven years. But by then DeBakey had mellowed to some extent: he was seventy-seven and still running Methodist Hospital like a military dictatorship. And he was still performing surgery, much to the dismay of several associates. But after being widowed in 1972, he remarried in 1975 to a stunning German actress by the name of Katrin Fehlhaber, whom he'd met at a party at the home of comedian and grateful patient Jerry Lewis. A sometime painter, Katrin journeyed to Houston to paint DeBakey's portrait and stayed. Maybe ten years of marriage to a beautiful woman thirty-four years younger had softened DeBakey; at any rate, he reached out to Bud at the end of a presentation. By way of rapprochement, DeBakey pointed out an error of omission in Bud's speech, reminding him that "inattention to detail was the hallmark of mediocrity." With those words, Bud was forgiven all. It was a DeBakey form of forgiveness.

Moreover, it became clear that the two needed each other. The head of the NHLBI was a Reagan administration appointee named Claude Lenfant, a spindly, balding Frenchman who was not a fan of the artificial heart. His stated reasons made perfect sense. He wanted to put more healthcare dollars into prevention, and believed that left ventricular assist devices were a better bet than a total artificial heart. Lenfant believed that successful research on that front would lead to more discoveries for a total artificial heart down the road.

But there was another rationale making the rounds at the time, which was that Lenfant's own plan for an artificial heart had suffered an early death at the hands of Willem Kolff. Whatever the truth—maybe a little of both—the artificial heart looked like it was heading for the junk heap of bad ideas.

Something else happened around that time that convinced the American people that bold experiments weren't such a great idea: on January 28, 1986, the space shuttle *Challenger* exploded seventy-three seconds into its tenth flight, killing all seven crew members aboard, including the first civilian to venture into space, a thirty-seven-year-old teacher named Christa McAuliffe. The disaster occurred in the late morning; like the Kennedy assassination, people spent the next few days glued to their television sets in horror and mourning, watching the rocket break into pieces again and again. (One study showed that about 17 percent of the country saw the launch, and the news spread to 85 percent of the population within an hour.) The shuttle program was mothballed for nearly three years, while a special commission appointed by President Reagan investigated the cause, and found the once heroic NASA culture severely wanting.

So maybe it wasn't surprising that the artificial heart—another technological gamble—would find its future threatened at around the same time. In May, Lenfant, acting alone, abruptly canceled the program, around the same time the Texas Heart Institute and four other institutions were due to receive approximately $22 million in NIH research contracts.

Maybe Lenfant should have thought things through a little more carefully. His action ignited a congressional battle that raged over the next few months like a wildfire out of control. Like so many political battles, this one had the veneer of high-mindedness—medical innovation that could save future lives versus medical innovation that took dollars away from other healthcare crises—with pragmatic, mostly economic concerns lurking underneath. Funding for the burgeoning AIDS crisis, too long ignored by the federal government, was certainly a factor.

Lenfant had a strong ally in the *New York Times*, which published a May 1988 editorial calling the artificial heart the "Dracula of medical technology" ("During its 24-year life this Dracula of a program sucked $240 million out of the National Heart, Lung and Blood Institute. At long last, the institute has found the resolve to drive a stake through its voracious creation"). That summer, the *Times* published an even more damning piece called "The Promise That Failed": "Our need to vanquish death has brought to center stage a new cultural archetype: Dirty Harrys with scalpels who have little patience for bureaucrats and ethical subtleties," wrote the author, Ralph Brauer, a conservative analyst with the Hubert Humphrey Institute of Public Affairs. The glamour of heart surgeons was fading fast: Ben Casey had morphed into Clint Eastwood's Hollywood detective who challenged bad guys to "make my day" by giving him an excuse to shoot to kill.

The pounding from the *Times*—and support for Lenfant—continued into July: "The artificial heart represents medical technology at its most mindless." And so on.

Two senators had the power to reverse Lenfant's decision, because they controlled the committee that oversaw funding for the National Institutes of Health: Ted Kennedy and Orrin Hatch, a Democrat and a Republican, who also happened to represent two states, Massachusetts and Utah, that had universities and companies with major investments in artificial heart R&D. That was how Bud wound up in Kennedy's office, essentially arguing against his boss at the NHLBI. Bud didn't dislike Lenfant—in fact, he was rather fond of him. He loved imitating his French accent. But Bud didn't like rules changed by fiat, especially when he felt the person making the rules didn't know what he was talking about and didn't try to find out by consulting anyone who was actually working in the field or who happened to be on his advisory committee. Like Bud Frazier.

So now Bud happily joined the fray, arguing democracy versus federalism—probably at length—with a pretty young aide in Kennedy's office. Bud was joined in the trenches with Robert Jarvik, who took on Lenfant and the *Times*, claiming, essentially, that both were un-American and maybe murderers too. "There is practically no Government money available for new concepts that can apply the extensive knowledge we have gained," Jarvik wrote in response to one of the negative editorials. "Thus the Government's program is barely limping along while heart disease remains our No. 1 killer. Dr. Lenfant's lack of urgency and leadership is disgraceful."

His arms sufficiently twisted—by congressional heavies more than by Jarvik and Frazier—Lenfant backed down in mid-July and restored the funding. "We felt the Heart Institute better eat a little crow rather than risk the future budgets of all the institutes," an NIH official confessed, not for attribution.

Bud Frazier went back to the THI, and back to work, his coffers replenished.

—∿—

It was a credit to Bud's obsessiveness—or his West Texas stubbornness, or his sometimes fritzy connection with the real world—that he persisted with his faith in continuous flow, despite the opposition from his colleagues. But there was another reason as well. In 1986, at a medical conference, two radically different men had approached him who supported his idea. In fact, they had been working independently on pulseless devices themselves. One was an engineer and heart surgeon by the name of Richard Wampler; the other was Robert Jarvik. Jarvik didn't know Wampler, and Wampler didn't know Jarvik. Wampler knew Frazier pretty much by reputation alone, while Jarvik and Frazier's relationship was like those couples who couldn't live with or without each other. Yes, most heart surgeons and cardiologists were pretty sure Frazier's pulseless heart notion was nuts. But everyone also knew that if you had wanted to explore something new in terms of the human heart, Bud was just about the only researcher to see, which was why Wampler and Jarvik sought him out.

Like Denton Cooley, Richard Wampler had always been an irrepressible tinkerer, the kid who fixed broken lawn mowers in his neighborhood in Bloomington, Indiana. When he was a boy, Wampler's beloved grandfather died of heart disease. The sense of helplessness he felt at his grandfather's bedside, while the doctors and nurses were shocking him with paddles trying to save his life, spurred him toward a career in medicine and also toward the belief that an artificial heart was not just possible but necessary. Maybe, he thought, he was the person who might be able to invent it.

Wampler was not a world-beater in the conventional sense. A classic midwesterner with soulful blue eyes, he was unflappable and wry. He also had a sense of adventure and a sense of obligation that found him in a small Egyptian village called El Bayad in 1976. Wampler was on a volunteer mission to help villagers improve their water supply. One day he saw two men using a submersible pump to draw water from Nile canals into their fields for irrigation. Because he was an engineer, and an expert on pumps, Wampler recognized this long tube with an internal, narrow corkscrew as an Archimedes' screw. Named after the third-century Greek mathematician, it worked like a plumber's augur. With the turn of a crank, water could be scooped from a lower place and forced to flow upward to another spot.

Not many people would have thought that such a pump might

be useful in treating heart disease, but most people did not see the world the way Wampler did. Like Bud's, his mind rarely strayed far from the idea of fixing damaged hearts. And like Bud, he had come to believe that the current iterations of heart pumps weren't good enough. Even with recent improvements, they were difficult and tricky to implant, and therefore dangerous: a surgeon had to open a patient's chest and cut into the heart and the aorta to attach them. That glimpse of the Archimedes' screw suggested to Wampler that something much smaller could be implanted, eliminating the need for the potentially debilitating heart-lung machine and open-heart surgery. Wampler didn't envision a permanent replacement for the heart or any of its parts—just something that could temporarily take over some of the functions of a weakened heart's pumping action. Other surgeons were beginning to look into continuous-flow pumps as well, like Leonard Golding at the Cleveland Clinic, but mostly the field was wide open, kind of like a plot of land in outer space.

Wampler went back to his home in Northern California and began designing and building a prototype for a new kind of heart pump—one that could help the heart move blood through the body by spinning instead of pumping. Initially, Wampler set up shop in the family kitchen, and began casting prototypes out of wax, like a jeweler. Fairly soon after, Wampler quit his job as an emergency room doctor and founded a medical device company that included a handful of aerospace engineers. He convinced them to work with him on a rotary pump, a device commonly used in everything from oil to milk production—anything that keeps liquids spinning continuously.

Wampler's group reflected his personality: they were true believers, dedicated, open-minded, and not in the least preoccupied with the business side of the enterprise. At least two hard-and-fast medical truths suggested that success was probably not in the cards: the first was the as yet undisputed belief that blood was very fragile and that spinning it at high speed would certainly destroy it, like fruit in a blender. The second was the conventional wisdom that heart disease could not be reversed. Once there was severe damage to the most vital of all organs, the end was ensured.

Nonetheless, Wampler gave his design specifications to a retired engineer who designed liquid hydrogen pumps for missiles. "Does this require a redefinition of the laws of physics or can this be done?" Wampler asked him. He had a hunch that if he could design a pump that spun fast enough, the blood would pass through safely, the way you can speed a finger through a candle flame.

The engineer agreed to give Wampler's idea a try, and soon came back to him with a working sketch and some calculations. Wampler then went to his workshop and fashioned the first blades out of mahogany, with a file and chisel. Eventually, after about a year, his team had something ready to test in calves. The device was remarkably small: the pump itself was encased in a titanium shell that fit easily in the palm of a hand. It was an axial pump, meaning it was long and extremely narrow, twice as long, in fact, as it was wide.

Essentially, it was a high-tech Archimedes' screw kept in place on either end by two magnetic bearings. Instead of carrying water for crops, it would—he hoped—ferry blood around the body. When Wampler began testing his device in the lab, he was surprised and encouraged to find that the bearings did not seem to crush blood as it flowed through the pump. What if the conventional wisdom was wrong?

As he had promised himself, Wampler greatly simplified the implantation process as well. His pump could be guided from the femoral artery in the leg up into the aortic valve—the valve between the aorta and the left ventricle—with the help of a fluoroscope. Once there, it could give a boost to a damaged left ventricle, which lacked enough blood to pump on its own.

At the time, there were no batteries or any other power source small enough to implant inside the body, so Wampler devised a motor that attached to the cable on the outside of a patient's leg as the power source.

It was around this time that Wampler, then forty, decided he was ready to reach out to a surgeon. And the surgeon who came highly recommended was named Bud Frazier. When Wampler finally contacted him at that fateful conference in 1986, Bud turned the device over in his hands, listening to Wampler's explanation. Then he told him it would never work. Sure, he believed in a pulseless pump, but he was also pretty sure that a pump spinning as fast as Wampler's would destroy the blood cells and lead to certain death. Still, he agreed to try the pump in a few calves.

That's when weird things started happening. The calves who were implanted didn't die right away. In fact, they lived long enough to suggest that Wampler's invention would work just the way he'd envisioned—not forever, but long enough to keep patients alive until they could get a transplant.

Bud became like a man who had found religion—or, maybe, like a man who now had proof that the God he'd never quite trusted actually existed. He started giving talks on the success of Wampler's pump. This could be it: a left ventricular assist device that was small and self-contained, with the kind of engineering that might later be applied to total artificial hearts. "We all thought that a pump spinning at 2,500 rpms would destroy the blood cells," he said in his first talk. "But we were wrong."

The ever-polite Wampler, who had been listening from the back of the room, waited until Bud was done before taking him aside to correct one small mistake in his talk. The pump actually spun at *25,000 rpm*, not 2,500, he said. Bud looked at Wampler as if he had been kicked by a mule. "If you'd told me that before, I never would have tried it," he said.

Still, neither Wampler nor Frazier was sure the animal tests told them much of anything about the success of the pump in humans. ("You just don't find cows with hardening of the arteries," was the way Wampler put it.) Eventually Bud recommended two patients who, as Wampler and Bud both recalled, had no chance of survival, so if the pump failed, Bud wouldn't have to feel guilty. The two doctors then got FDA approval for emergency use and got the hospital's permission to operate, and Wampler shipped down an operating console while hand-carrying the pump to Houston himself. When he met up with Bud again, Wampler was unnerved to see Bud wearing cowboy boots. Was this guy really okay?

The patient ultimately chosen was a sixty-two-year-old Colorado man named Herb Kranich. Kranich had the weathered skin of the Colorado outdoorsman he once had been. He had silver hair, twinkling eyes under thick dark brows, and a warm, stoic nature. But he was a goner. He had had a transplant a month before, and his body was rejecting it by the minute; at this point he was pale, bedridden, and barely able to breathe, much less communicate. "If you've been in clinical medicine awhile, you can tell when someone is circling the drain," Wampler said.

Decades later, Wampler could clearly recall the stream of thoughts that flowed swiftly through his mind when he and Bud went in to ask Kranich's wife, Leslie, for permission to operate. "Your husband is going to die, and we know you are desperate—but we have this idea that has worked pretty well on cows . . . but we've never used it on a patient, here are two or three pages of complications, and in all honesty there's probably another page of complications, we just don't even know what they are yet. So what do you think? Do you want us to try?" Wampler was stunned when she agreed. Leslie Kranich felt that her husband had been so sick, and in and out of hospitals so much, that they had to go for broke. "This isn't living," she told the doctors.

Bud rushed Kranich into surgery on April 26, 1988—taking a little time off from the national artificial heart debate still raging in Washington. The actual operation took only twenty minutes or so. Inserting the cable on a course through Kranich's body turned out to be a lot easier than navigating the vicissitudes of Congress. Bud positioned the device—christened the Hemopump—in the aortic valve, and waited. He did not have to wait long, because it started working right away. Within twenty-four hours, the color returned to Kranich's face, his breathing became less labored, his blood gases rose, his fingers warmed. He was returned to life, even though he had only the faintest pulse; instead, there was the soft rushing sound of his blood spinning through the pump, which was pushing three or so liters through Kranich's body; five was normal, but for a man on bed rest, three would do just fine.

Within a few months, Herb Kranich was able to pack his bags and leave St. Luke's Hospital to return home to his family. There was no reason for a longer stay. The Hemopump demonstrated what DeBakey had suspected back in 1963: that given help and time to rest, the heart could sometimes recover on its own. Wampler and Frazier, neither of whom was given to hyperbole, were confounded. Heart failure, it turned out, didn't have to be a death sentence. They had also upended what doctors thought they knew about the blood, which had turned out to be a lot less fragile than previously be-lieved. Both men would say that witnessing Kranich's miraculous recovery was one of the most astonishing experiences of their lives. As Wampler would later say, "It convinced me that these perceived barriers were not barriers. The paradigms are very powerful, even if they are totally wrong."

Indeed, the Hemopump looked like nothing short of a medical miracle, and it was covered as such by the *Los Angeles Times* and the *New York Times*. *Discover* magazine called the device one of the 100 best inventions of the year. Even the *National Enquirer* featured it on the cover, next to game-show eye candy Vanna White. Wampler and Frazier were celebrities at the next ASAIO meeting; even Kolff made a point of congratulating them. If no side effects were discovered in future operations, Bud believed, the temporary pump could save as many as 150,000 lives a year.

There were, of course, more hurdles before the Hemopump could be used that way. Most crucial was winning FDA approval, which demanded extensive and stringent clinical trials for life-sustaining devices like the Hemopump, which were ranked in the strictest category. A recent scandal involving a defective and deadly heart valve meant the federal agency was even more vigilant than usual. The prospect of widows testifying in tears before a congressional committee wasn't good for anyone except plaintiffs' lawyers. The era of medical malpractice and product liability lawsuits was by then well established. The inventor of the Hemopump also had to show that the medical device could be commercially reproducible—safely—on a mass scale. Many companies came courting—what business wouldn't be interested in a device that could promise to commute the death sentence of at least 150,000 people overnight?

At first, things went well. Wampler's original company, Nimbus, raised enough capital to move forward. Seventy centers were set up to implant the Hemopump, and more than a hundred patients were saved. But over time, operating and production issues crept in, which did not sit well with officials at the FDA. The Hemopump wasn't a simple medical device, like a syringe or a tongue depressor. It took highly skilled teams to implant and monitor it, and sufficiently qualified people were not used often enough. So the pumps started failing. Suddenly Wampler found himself shuttling to Washington, trying to explain his device and its problems to anxious young bureaucrats who were not in the medical field, much less experts on blood pumps. He would try to dumb down his presentations but knew the officials were in over their heads. He could sense what was coming. FDA regulators were not risk takers by nature or by training; the penalty for approving a medical device that could fail—that is, kill people—was severe.

In the early 1990s, the FDA refused to grant free market approval, which meant Nimbus could not market the Hemopump commercially. The CEO suggested an IPO to raise more money for new trials, but the Nimbus board wouldn't approve it. They didn't want to dilute their ownership of what they knew was a miracle device. Instead, as Wampler would say, they got 100 percent of nothing.

Johnson & Johnson bought the technology and hired Wampler as a consultant, but ultimately the complexity of the product defeated them. They sold the Hemopump to Medtronics, another large medical device company. The pumps were cheap—$3,000 or so—but hospitals just wouldn't bite when told they had to make an expensive, up-front investment on the operating console.

The Hemopump was as good as dead, commercially. Medtronics buried their surplus consoles in a landfill, and with them Rich Wampler's dreams.

SYNCHRONICITY

There is an aspect of medical progress, or probably progress in any field, that has to do with something indefinable in the air, a breeze that only a select few can feel against their skin. Bud likes to cite a mass-market movie released in 1981 called *Threshold*, which starred Jeff Goldblum as a nerdy inventor and Donald Sutherland as a Cooley-type surgeon, both of whom become obsessed with creating an artificial heart. The screenwriter was James Salter, who, along with producing great novels like *A Sport and a Pastime*, also wrote a pre–Barney Clark profile of Robert Jarvik and covered the Akutsu implantation with Cooley in 1981 for *Life*.

To see *Threshold* today is a little eerie. It isn't a very good movie, but the characters speak authoritatively about technology that had not yet been invented. Actors use the term "continuous flow," for instance, long before Bud Frazier and a few colleagues started using the term to describe an alternative to the heart's pulsations. The movie also came out before Barney Clark got his Jarvik-7 and long before the *Challenger* explosion—that is, before the American public's faith in science and technology started to slip.

Sutherland did some of his research for the role at THI, and does a pretty good if somewhat severe impression of Cooley, who in the film is tortured because he cannot save his patients from dying of heart disease. (Cooley let Sutherland do a few stitches on a patient to get into his role, and makes a cameo appearance in the movie.) The basis for Goldblum's on-the-spectrum character is harder to pinpoint, but some of his awkwardness and obsessiveness is reminiscent of Robert Jarvik. The only thing that seems far too optimistic is the (not uncommon) premise that the artificial heart is just a few years away: Mare Winningham, playing a teenager who nearly dies of heart failure, walks out of the hospital under her own power, her mechanical heart whirring in her chest, no strings or wires or battery packs attached. You'd never even know she had one.

Bud still shakes his head in wonder at the movie, which he's seen more than a few times. How a Hollywood screenwriter could imagine a notion that he was just beginning to conjure still amazes him. "The actors even said things I've said," he likes to say, and it's true. The funny thing about the real development of continuous flow and its effect on artificial heart development is that it is far more entertaining and fluky than *Threshold* suggests, at least from that day in Louisville in 1986 when Bud encountered both Rich Wampler and Rob Jarvik.

Wampler's approach to Bud was straightforward because he is a straightforward man. Jarvik's approach reflected his personality too. He took Bud into a corner, where he surreptitiously opened a small package to show Bud the contents. The way Bud tells it, Jarvik acted like a person does "when you were in old Mexico and someone said they had pictures of naked girls—'Hey, come 'ere, señor.' Rob didn't want anybody to see it even then." The moment was a turning point for Bud: two total strangers picked up on the same idea—building a nonpulsatile heart pump—and then separately came to him because he was the best person to do the lab experiments that would make their idea a reality. Put another way, he was the only person with the clinical expertise and the lab resources who did not think the idea was a ludicrous, hopeless waste of time and money.

Jarvik, like Wampler, had come up with a tiny heart assist pump—an LVAD—that used continuous flow instead of pulsations. It was an axial pump, about the shape and size of a C battery, with a mechanism like an Archimedes' screw. The difference between the two was that Jarvik's heart, unlike Wampler's, was designed not as a temporary device but as a permanent one.

Bud studied the pump as well as he could, given Jarvik's furtiveness, and agreed to try it on some animals in his lab. How was it that Wampler and Jarvik, two men who had never met, came up with the same idea at the same time? No one knows. There had been some debate already about pulseless devices, and some hypothetical papers written. And guys with engineering and design backgrounds were probably among the most likely to catch the breeze.

There was one other notable difference between the two men: Robert Jarvik was more difficult to deal with than Richard Wampler.

When Bud reflects on his decades-long relationship with Jarvik, he sounds like someone talking about a difficult family member who wouldn't be missed at Thanksgiving dinner. The two spent several years paired on various medical panels at various conferences around the world. Bud had pegged Jarvik as "a chatterbox." It annoyed him that Jarvik never missed a chance to one-up everybody else, including him. Whenever he came to Houston, Jarvik always wanted to go to chi-chi restaurants that Bud wasn't interested in. Sometimes Bud would say, explaining his relationship, "I was one of the few people who could get along with Jarvik," and at other times he would say, "I never really got along with Jarvik very well," or "Rob is hard to like," depending on where they were in their relationship. The truth is that they were lashed together by mutual interest. Both were determined to come up with a total artificial heart, which probably made working together simultaneously more collegial and more fraught. Jarvik knew how to make devices, and Bud knew how they would work in the body and had the best lab for testing them. Neither man, however, was particularly skilled at give-and-take.

Still, there was a lot more tolerance among the community of heart surgeons for Bud, partly because he *was* a heart surgeon, and an accomplished one, and also because he was just a nicer guy. Bud can suck the air out of the room as well as or better than anybody, but you also feel that if you really *had* to tell a story of your own, he would at least try to listen. And, of course, if you were sick, you could be absolutely sure that he would sit by your bedside until the sun came up and went down again.

Jarvik, on the other hand, is not a heart surgeon and never practiced medicine; he belongs to no fraternity and has never seemed to care in the least about joining one. He is an inventor first and foremost, and not at all what you would call a people person. In fact, Jarvik often radiates a kind of weary boredom, unless he is demonstrating something he has invented; then his personality and passion bloom as he offers lots of eye contact while casually caressing his device in a way that is almost erotic. He has the bust of a mannequin in his office that is outfitted with something that looks like a cochlear implant. In fact, it is a heart assist device in which a power cable is snaked from the pump through the neck and connected to a skull-mounted pedestal behind the ear. When Jarvik starts talking about design and function, caressing the dummy's head with his long, delicate fingers, your thoughts might wander to that part of the book of Genesis where God makes man.

On that fateful day Jarvik showed Bud his super-secret pump, an LVAD that would come to be known as the Jarvik 2000, things were not going so well. The board of the company he had founded to market the Jarvik-7, Symbion, had invested $40 million and had little to show for it. Symbion was becoming a takeover target because it was badly managed—some would say by Jarvik himself. (He would be fired by the board within the year, with a $3 million payout.) "Jarvik was run out of Utah," is the way Bud put it. He moved to Manhattan, but kept working with William DeVries, the surgeon who had implanted the heart in Barney Clark. Having shifted his base of operations to Louisville, Kentucky, DeVries' work on artificial hearts was now underwritten by Humana, the giant for-profit healthcare conglomerate.

The good and bad news was that this was the tightfisted, authoritarian era of managed care. Humana, often portrayed in the media as the biggest villain on the healthcare block for denying care, was in need of a little positive PR of its own. The corporation became just the angel Jarvik and DeVries needed when it agreed to underwrite one hundred artificial heart implants at an estimated cost of $25 million.

The four Jarvik-7 hearts implanted at the Humana Heart Institute in 1984 and 1985 were not viewed as successes. Most patients died within a matter of months. The longest survivor was William Schroeder, who lived nearly two years but endured multiple strokes and other debilitating conditions, all of which were recorded by the press. Instead of being a poster boy for the artificial heart, Schroeder became another living argument against medical progress for the sake of medical progress.

Life magazine's May 1985 story on Schroeder sported a hopeful cover: DeVries, fit and beaming, posed with a protective arm around him. The patient wore an oxygen tube protruding from his nose, and the distracted smile of someone who wasn't quite there. The subtitle inside was far less optimistic than previous artificial heart coverage: "The Troubling Story Behind a Historic Experiment." The story itself was pretty negative too.

None of this reflected well on Jarvik. It wasn't exactly his fault that the media had tried to fashion him as another medical superstar in the tradition of Barnard, Cooley, or DeBakey. But Jarvik was ill-suited to the role. Although he looked the part—Jarvik was indisputably handsome, even sexy, especially when photographers enticed him to pose in a motorcycle jacket or shirtless. But his personality didn't lend itself to the all-access journalism of the time. Up close, Jarvik wasn't nearly as suave as he appeared, even when he posed as an iconic, eye-patch-wearing man in the Hathaway shirt. By the mid-eighties, his own negatives and the negatives about the artificial heart were overlapping like crashing waves in a gathering storm.

A case in point was a *Playboy* profile published in April 1986. It's hard to believe in retrospect, but at the time submitting to a *Playboy* profile, like participating in the *Playboy* Interview, was a mark of distinction, even though everyone knew that the real purpose of the journalism in the magazine was to serve as intellectual cover for all those foldouts of young and very buxom naked women. Still, the exposure was probably irresistible to Jarvik, as it had been for Frank Sinatra, Fidel Castro, Vladimir Nabokov, Ingmar Bergman, Elisabeth Kübler-Ross, Lech Walesa, Jimmy Carter, and so many others.

But, as many celebrities would soon learn, there *was* such a thing as bad publicity. "The Rock and Roll Heart of Robert Jarvik" homed in on the subject's complete obliviousness to normal human conduct, such as Jarvik's laser-like determination over a weekend with the writer's family to build a dildo in the shape of a unicorn horn for a new lady friend. As in: "The ovens were heating up for dinner, and we were about to begin when Jarvik insisted that his dildo be baked first . . . we all stood around for half an hour—my wife, my parents, two of my hungry brothers and I . . . until Dr. Jarvik declared it finished."

This kind of behavior made it increasingly difficult for Jarvik to find colleagues and funding for future projects. Bud was, in essence, the safest and last resort.

When Bud inspected Jarvik's device, he had one major suggestion. The pump should go inside the left ventricle, instead of fitting outside the heart and under the diaphragm, like most of the LVADs then in use. That way, there would be less crowding inside the torso and less discomfort—and, more important, less chance of infection. At the time, surgeons had to make something called a "pump pocket" to fit the pumps in, but those pockets were perfect receptacles for bacteria and, eventually, infections.

But putting the pump inside the ventricle itself created problems of its own. Jarvik's pump, like Wampler's, used bearings at either end of the rotor. Wherever a moving part comes into contact with a non-moving part, a bearing is needed as a transition; otherwise, the connecting points will literally grind to a halt. But bearings need lubrication to do their job. The bearings that kept the rotor turning inside Wampler's pump were lubricated with a glucose solution via a line from outside the body. But you couldn't have a line like that going directly into the heart if your device was supposed to be totally implantable.

Jarvik had a solution for that problem: using the blood flowing through the pump to provide the lubrication. This was like declaring that soapy water would work as well as motor oil in a car. It didn't sound like a workable idea. And, of course, this was in the mid-1980s, when almost everyone still believed that blood was as fragile in a centrifugal pump as an overheated southern belle on the dance floor. Medical experts felt Jarvik's design, like Wampler's, was doomed because the bearings would crush the blood as it passed through, destroying red blood cells, and so on until death.

Bud, however, was intrigued. Jarvik might be a pain in the ass, but he was very good at making things—in fact, no one in the biomedical field was better. And unlike Wampler, Jarvik already had a prototype for a pulseless/continuous-flow device. So Bud agreed to give the pump a try in a few poor calves.

There was, however, a bigger problem: money. Jarvik didn't have any and wasn't willing to trust his creation to venture capitalists, given his experience with Symbion. And government grants for an artificial heart, by this time, were about as rare as self-effacing heart surgeons.

That is when Bud, who had a vested interest in proving the merit of continuous flow, came up with a novel solution. For years his department had earned $2,000 each time someone went to pick up a donor heart for transplantation—in the early days, Bud was the doctor charged with flying to a designated hospital and cutting the heart out of a brain-dead donor. ("It's a ten-minute operation. You just have to know where to cut and put the heart in an ice pack and get back on the plane.") Having never been obsessed with money, Bud at first refused it and then just put each fee in a fund for the THI lab and forgot about it. But Cooley's booming transplant program had been an unexpected boon—by the time Jarvik approached him, Bud had about $50,000 put away. That was enough to use on a few experiments.

Thus began a process that was slow-moving and not very encouraging. There were no software programs at the time for designing much of anything, much less artificial hearts. Jarvik made the titanium pump himself—doing all the drawing, cutting, sanding, and polishing. His goal was to make something small enough to fit inside the heart but strong enough to push blood through the thousands of vessels in the body.

Jarvik insisted on scrubbing in on the implantations in the lab. It both amused and appalled the others present to see him peering over the great Dr. Frazier's shoulder, enjoying the privilege of calling him Bud when the rest of the team wouldn't dare, suggesting he move the pump up a little, or down a little, or a little toward the left or right. You could almost see the thought bubbles over everyone's head: Jarvik had never practiced medicine. Jarvik was not a surgeon, much less a THI surgeon. Who did this guy think he was? Bud, though, chuckled and responded like a teacher indulging an eager if misguided child.

The result of the first animal implant was probably predictable: within three days, the pump froze, and the calf died. A technician in Bud's lab removed the pump and sent it back to New York, where Jarvik made changes in his design, particularly in the bearings, which he deemed to be the problem. This went on for the next few *years*. Jarvik would study what he had done before, make more adjustments in the bearings, and send a new pump to Houston. That pump would then go in a calf, and the calf would live a little bit longer, but never quite long enough. Something about the shape, size, or polishing of the bearings was always off. After several years, Jarvik was almost ready to give up on the idea.

Not that all was lost. By August 1987, Jarvik had divorced his wife and left his two children in Utah to move to New York, where he married Marilyn Vos Savant, a dark-haired stunner who made a name for herself as the Smartest Woman in the World. Vos Savant claimed to have the highest IQ of anyone on the planet, which won her not just the Smartest Man on the Planet but an advice column called "Ask Marilyn" in the Sunday supplement *Parade*. (You were supposed to ask her tough questions about math and probability, such as "Are men smarter than women?") She parlayed that success into book contracts for tomes that promised to make readers as smart as she was. The couple shared an apartment on the West Side of the city, where Vos Savant wrote and Jarvik had his lab. According to one publication, they spent a lot of time discussing the nature of reality.

It was the success of the Hemopump in 1988 that finally

galvanized Jarvik—specifically, it was Wampler's discovery that blood could spin at high speeds without damage. By 1989 or 1990, Jarvik had figured out that the difference between a pump that worked and one that didn't had to do with the way he was polishing the bearings. As it turned out, the difference between a bearing that worked and a bearing that failed was a difference that could only be measured in microns.

By then, the calves were living eight months with his pump, well past the FDA requirement to begin human trials. Bud noticed that they had gotten so big they were leaving giant hoof prints on the floor of the lab.

Then they faced another hurdle. FDA trials, as Wampler had learned, were expensive and risky. Jarvik would need to pay for personnel, testing, and so on. But unlike Wampler, he continued to refuse to work with any venture capitalists. A solution seemed to come from the federal government: the Small Business Administration, under George H. W. Bush, was giving out loans to encourage growth, including loans to companies that made medical devices. Jarvik was nothing if not a small businessman, and so he applied.

Unfortunately, the person charged with approving the loans in the medical field was Michael DeBakey, who was not a member of the Robert Jarvik fan club. Even though members of his committee recommended funding the pump, DeBakey turned the Jarvik application down flat.

Then something really odd happened. DeBakey—who had never reopened his artificial heart lab after the Cooley/Liotta betrayal—came out with a pump that was also continuous flow, with bearings lubricated by blood. According to DeBakey, the device had been developed over a period of years with the help of NASA engineers. But to people around THI at the time, the DeBakey pump was strikingly similar to Jarvik's—and debuted very soon after Jarvik had submitted his detailed schematics to DeBakey's committee for the small business loan.

Jarvik was so upset that in a phone call he told Bud he was thinking of suing.

DeBakey, however, wasn't rattled. "I don't know what stage his device is in," he told a reporter around that time. "I'm sure that he's trying to compete too."

DeBakey certainly moved faster. He arranged to have his pump implanted in a patient in Europe in 1998. (By this time, inventors were doing their testing outside the United States because FDA requirements had become so constraining that it was virtually impossible to adhere to them.) Bud was not impressed with some aspects of the design, and indeed, with more implantations, the pump caused an excessive number of strokes. If that wasn't bad enough, the company formed to market the pump was bought by a hedge fund that was soon embroiled in a financial scandal—and not long afterward abandoned DeBakey, his company, and his pump.

This should have given Jarvik some satisfaction—along with the fact that his pump worked a lot better than its supposed twin. Bud implanted it in a middle-aged woman named Lois Spiller in 2000, who thrived—Jarvik had even added a dial that could be adjusted to increase blood flow. "When I get tired I just turn those numbers up and I can walk some more," Spiller told her surgeon, Bud Frazier.

But fate intervened again. Cardiologists and surgeons did not like the Jarvik 2000 because they didn't want to work with Jarvik. Meanwhile, Jarvik hadn't kept good enough records to submit to the FDA to complete his trial, and Bud's records were destroyed in a Houston flood in 2001. So the Jarvik 2000, a fully implantable heart assist device, has yet to be approved for use by the government. Bud calls it, "the longest FDA trial in history."

There was, however, another pulseless, implantable device that seemed to hold a lot of promise around that time. Bud's old partner Vic Poirier of Thoratec had been working with Rich Wampler on a new iteration of the Hemopump, called the HeartMate II. In 2008, it won FDA approval as a bridge to transplant, and two years later it was approved for long-term use.

As Robert Jarvik told a reporter in a slightly different context, referencing DeBakey, "If you compare it to a prize fight, who throws the punch first is not so important as who's there at the end and who throws the punch last."

THE KING OF DISTRACTION

One of the few things Billy Cohn loved as much as working as a Texas Heart Institute heart surgeon was Halloween. If he were self-aware—and he could be, at times—he might have noted that celebrating the holiday on a grand scale allowed him to combine many of the things he loved: magic, performance, and making something with his preternaturally active hands. A person with normal levels of time and creativity would have to sacrifice something to prepare for what was, for Billy, a suburban-scale spectacle, but he possessed one of those minds that could either (a) contain many thoughts, plans, and ideas at once or (b) move so fast it just seemed that way. Billy was a raffishly handsome man with a nasal Houston twang—blue-eyed, reddish-blond hair thinning into a precise widow's peak, a sharp nose, and a cock-of-the-walk stride. He favored inky black cowboy boots with his scrubs, and was best taken at face value.

In other words, the Great Halloween Extravaganza of 2013 didn't take away from Billy's very busy life as a surgeon and inventor, or, for that matter, from his obsessive sidelines as musician and magician. Billy played trombone in a number of bands around town, usually on weekdays in the late evenings, often after surgery. He was also

a master of card tricks, punctuating many a slow (for Billy) dinner with his favorite sleight of hand, converting five one-dollar bills
into five $100 bills. Billy was also married and a father of five chil-
dren, each of whom in some way reflected their father's energy and/
or talents, as if his personality had been fractured into his progeny
like a beam of light shot through a prism. In contrast, Billy's wife,
Mishaun, a stay-at-home mom who is also a card-carrying member
of Mensa, displayed an uncanny ability to go along to get along, the
only way a person could probably live with Billy for any extended
period of time.

The Cohn mansion in the once modest but now substantially
upgraded neighborhood of Bellaire resembled Tara from the outside,
including the obligatory columns and porticoes. Inside, it looked a
little like the place had been recently ransacked, with several generations of toys and games and electrical equipment throughout. Things
went missing, like the top to the toilet tank. This made repairs easier
when the thing kept running, because you could just reach in and
pull the float up by hand.

Billy's workshop out back, behind the expansive patio and pool
and the vintage Jaguar with leopard-spotted upholstery parked under
the porte cochere, was in a similar state. There were metal shelves
and pegboards that looked post-implosion, with countless hanging
and tangled wires and tubes, adhesives, straps, and other assorted
unidentifiable (to anyone but Billy) objects. Creations, partial and
complete, dangled from pegboards. A poster for a new kind of surgical needle Billy had invented featured a multiply pierced hipster with
the caption "Too Many Holes?" He could have been Billy, back in
his punk-rocker phase.

The workshop was the place Billy retreated when he needed to
focus, and he needed to focus for Halloween. This year's concept had
been percolating in his mind for quite some time—a week or so. The
Bellaire house had a sprawling front lawn, punctuated at the curb by

two large oaks. A distance of about twenty feet separated the house from the trees, a span that suggested to Billy some form of transport. Aerial transport.

Coincidentally, Billy had come across one of his nineteen-year-old daughter's abandoned dolls. Its silky yellow hair had turned ratty from affection and overuse, and suggested at least one encounter with, maybe, electrocution. The doll's white lace dress, once pristine, starched and neatly banded with pink satin, was now dingy with age, the color of bad teeth.

Over the next few days, Billy added bright red stains and mud-colored spots to the dress. He painted the top half of her face death-bed white, while the bottom half he made as red as arterial blood. Ditto her right arm. He fiddled with her body, moving the arms and legs up and down until the doll assumed the position of a superhero flying through the air. He strung wires from the trees to his front door, and motorized the whole thing with a remote-control box he adapted from one of his sons' toy cars. By Halloween, his creation was ready to go.

Like virtually every Billy Cohn invention, this one was a big success. Here they'd come, the wide-eyed, mega-coddled innocents of Bellaire, the ones whose mothers walked them into school every day and baked gluten-free classroom cookies. Or the kids in Freddy Krueger masks and polyester Disney princess costumes from the apartment complexes in nearby Gulfton, chattering away in Spanish. They'd skip up the Cohn driveway, their sacks already open, greedy for candy, and then—out of nowhere—this screeching doll would swoop down on them, grazing their tiny scalps like a hungry, furious, completely crazed madgirl.

It did take a while to calm the kids down, but then they went scrambling through the house to Cohn's second-floor balcony to watch the next bunch of kids get tachycardia.

A cynic could suggest that Billy was creating his next generation of patients. Or that, despite his 24/7 schedule, he still couldn't keep himself busy.

—∿—

A lot of surgeons are satisfied just to be surgeons. Or even highly specialized surgeons, like neurosurgeons or cardiothoracic surgeons, Billy's chosen field. Most such super-specialists are happy enough to stand over a fully anesthetized human body and sew up a ruptured aorta while the seconds tick away and a life hangs perilously in the balance. Every damn day that kind of doctor gets up and at least tries to save a life—and the riskier the practice, the likelier the loss. Looking deep into the eyes of the desperate turned grateful, even worshipful—for most, that's enough. That and the exhilaration of beating the odds. Again.

So yes, Billy loved going to the Texas Heart Institute every morning. He couldn't believe he got to work alongside the men who had been his heroes and mentors, such as Denton Cooley and, now, Bud Frazier. Even so, he needed more. Billy wasn't unlike a very busy bee buzzing from flower to flower—all that pollen was delicious, but there never seemed to be enough of it. In that regard, he was lucky to have come into his own at a time when the medical profession was in something of a supercharged, if chaotic, phase. The doctor who made house calls or even one who sat at the foot of your hospital bed offering comfort and encouragement—like the iconic TV doc Marcus Welby or even, say, Michael DeBakey or Bud Frazier— was speedily going the way of the VCR and the landline. First there was all the paperwork demanded by the managed care experiment, and soon there would be the all-inclusive concierge care, where for around $2,000 a year, the wealthy could buy the bedside manner.

But at the same time, the medical world had expanded in ways that better suited someone like Billy, temperamentally, intellectually, and creatively.

Put another way, the medical and engineering professions were like a couple who were profoundly ill-suited for each other but determined to work together for the sake of the children. Yes, there were myriad inventions that had required joint efforts—the heart-lung machine being one of them—but the engineer and the physician rarely if ever sat down together, and then only when necessary. There were many theories for this conflict. One had to do with different training. Engineers were taught to be "divergent thinkers," to explore as many answers as possible when looking for a solution—like, say, bringing the astronauts home safely during the Apollo 13 disaster. Physicians, in contrast, were taught to be "convergent thinkers"—to believe that there was only one right answer to the way the body worked and you'd better know it in a crisis.

A somewhat conflicting theory held that medicine was for a very long time more of an art than a science, and engineering was rooted firmly in the concrete. Then too, doctors were sure they were smarter than engineers (and everyone else), and engineers thought they were smarter than doctors (and everyone else).

The rapid expansion and overwhelming intricacies of technology forced them together. With every increase in knowledge about the body, medicine became not just more specialized but more dependent on things that themselves had increased in complexity. Those advances made possible inventions that would have been unimaginable just a few decades ago: artificial titanium hips, flexible and pressure-sensitive artificial skin, micro-rockets that delivered medicine to just the right spot in the body, prosthetics operated from deep in the mind, and so on. No one person—even a surgeon! even an engineer!—could possibly keep up. Yes, Denton Cooley could build a precursor of a heart-lung machine with materials from the hardware store in the 1950s, but by the 1980s, few if any medical professionals could actually make a medical device that could be mass-produced and not only worked electronically—or with lasers or magnets or ten jillion computer data points—but could also pass muster with the FDA. (God help you if you got a pacemaker or a heart valve to market that then developed issues; as Rich Wampler and Robert Jarvik knew all too well, even the hint of a life-threatening problem would damn your invention to obscurity.)

And, then, thanks to the Barney Clark debacle and other medical failures—in particular the IUD—the great enthusiasm of the federal government for funding giant medical breakthroughs had declined significantly. This didn't mean there wasn't money to be had; it just meant that most of the money needed for medical research was now coming from private sources, venture capitalists who were more than willing to pour cash into a creative endeavor, as long as they got a huge piece of the action and it met with great success. Which didn't necessarily mean that it saved lives but rather that it generated hundreds of millions, or even billions, for its investors. Witness the disaster that was the Hemopump. Failure in medicine and medical innovation was as natural as life and death, but it was also not an option.

This was the world in which Billy Cohn came of age.

One of the most frequently repeated stories about Billy—and sometimes not by Billy himself—is that, growing up in the prosperous Memorial section of Houston's prosperous west side, his mother, Judy, would leave newspaper clippings about Michael DeBakey and

Denton Cooley beside his cereal bowl in the mornings. This move could be interpreted as a classic Jewish mother ploy (a Houston Jewish mother in particular), but it might also have been a vain attempt to keep Billy on the straight and narrow. By his admission—not his adoring mother's—Billy did not apply himself in elementary school, maybe because he had a touch of ADHD and maybe because he was just supremely bored because he was so smart. Or both. It is perhaps notable that his father, an advertising and marketing executive, came to Houston to work for the mildly certifiable Judge Roy Hofheinz to publicize the judge's new pro baseball team, the Colt .45s (soon to become the Astros), along with the eighth wonder of the world, the Astrodome, the nation's first indoor stadium. The Dome was, to say the least, a marvel of engineering and a perfect example of Thinking Big, Texas style, but in a good way.

Coincidentally or not—depending on how big a believer you were in Houston's possibilities—it was during this time that NASA was launching its manned spaceflight missions. During the sixties and seventies, Billy's parents were friendly with many of the astronauts, some of whom even came to dinner at the house. ("My family is manically extroverted," John Cohn, Billy's older brother, explained.) If you were a hypercreative boy in Houston during that time, it was pretty easy to believe you could do just about anything you set your mind to.

In fact, from a very early age, Billy and his brother, John, spent a lot of time unsupervised—their mother and father predated the age of helicopter parenting—and entranced with science experiments that mostly involved blowing things up in bigger and better ways. Their parents were extremely bright: mother Judy had been in Sylvia Plath's class at Smith, father Hugh was a self-starter who thrived as a marketing and advertising executive in the Mad Men era in Manhattan. "In our family you had to be sharp," John Cohn said. "To be half a step behind on a joke was almost unthinkable." Science was in the family genes: Billy's uncle, Arnall Patz, was the revered Johns Hopkins ophthalmologist who discovered the link between anesthesia and childhood blindness. At every holiday or birthday where gifts were exchanged, the Cohn brothers asked for chemistry sets. They built their own lab in the garage. They became potato cannon sharpshooters.

At this point, you might have expected Billy to take his rightful place in pocket protector nerddom, especially in a white-bread, deeply conformist suburb like Memorial. But several factors worked against that. He was a good-looking kid, blond and blue-eyed, quick-witted—often to the point of impatience—and less interested in book learning than in figuring things out on his own. He was good with his hands: Billy was one of those kids who could master almost anything he tried, who was able to intuit the mechanics of virtually any device he laid his eyes on. And, thanks to a dad in PR, he was also able to communicate to the mechanically challenged just what, exactly, he was doing and why. He was very popular.

Still, his mother worried that Billy was never quite able to settle on anything. In high school, he joined the marching band after teaching himself how to play the trombone. He also taught himself to play the guitar, electric and acoustic, and started playing in high school bands. He liked to draw, so he got himself a job designing and silk-screening T-shirts, and then another decorating cakes at Baskin-Robbins. Mostly he nurtured the nebulous goal of becoming a rock star. The punk scene was coming on strong, and it seemed a good fit for his musical and theatrical gifts as well as his psychological makeup.

Then he got to college at Oberlin. "I quickly saw that I didn't have to live up to anyone's expectations, that I didn't have to follow some already-in-place-plan for my life," he would say later. On the other hand, Billy's first career choice was looking like a non-starter.

Oberlin seemed full of musicians with rock-star dreams. Billy aced the MCAT—he had fortuitously completed a double major in biology and chemistry. Then, almost on the fly—he missed most medical school application deadlines—he applied to Baylor and several other med schools, and through what he himself says might have been divine intervention, along with a summer job with his mother's Baylor-trained doc, he got in. It is safe to say that Billy was the only med student there with a rainbow-hued punk 'do.

As it happened, the challenges and the demands of medicine appealed to him, as well as the intensity—the churning Ben Taub Hospital emergency room, one of the busiest in the nation, was the perfect place for a young, perpetually restless surgeon. As a cardiac surgery resident in 1991, Billy never had time for his mind to wander; the place wasn't nicknamed the "Houston Knife and Gun Club" for nothing. He was fast and thorough, and soon enough developed the been-through-the-fire Baylor swagger. Toward the end of his residency, Billy won the dubious honor of serving as Michael DeBakey's last chief resident. DeBakey, in his eighties, finally put his scalpel down in 1993, to the relief of many.

Like Bud, Billy intuited what he was supposed to be in DeBakey's presence—that is, perfect—and accepted the challenge, even though doing so meant hiding his eight hundred watts under the proverbial bushel while amping up his hypervigilant side. "You had to be smart and you had to be resilient because they would beat you down," his wife, Mishaun, explained. By then, Billy was accustomed to the abuse and the lack of sleep; now he read and memorized every page of patients' charts to avoid DeBakey's passion for humiliation. He became expert at dispensing the "proximity beating," following De-Bakey's predilection for screaming at whoever was closest to him for whatever went wrong, regardless of who was really at fault.

By the time Billy finished his surgical residency at Baylor, he was certain of one thing: he did not want to go into private practice. The idea of doing the same thing over and over again, day in and day out, was, for him, a form of torture. He applied for and won a coveted fellowship at Harvard Medical School, followed by a full-time faculty position and, eventually, a directorship of Minimally Invasive Surgery at the prestigious Beth Israel Deaconess Medical Center. Unable to give up his rock-star dreams, he also kept playing in bands in his off-hours.

It was during this time that Billy, like Denton Cooley, came to see that his constant tinkering could come to more. He had an unconscious, automatic compulsion that allowed him—drove him—to see and solve mechanical problems. Billy installed a metal shop in the basement of the small house he shared with his growing family in Brookline. (At that point, Billy and Mishaun had two children in diapers. Ostensibly, they weren't allowed in the basement.)

The first invention he brought to near completion was a portable blood warmer. Unfortunately, no one, even a highly trained engineer, could bring his idea to life at the time because the technology to keep the blood undamaged and at a steady temperature outside a hospital setting did not yet exist. (For hospital operations, blood is refrigerated and then warmed before transfusions for adequate circulation. If you were, say, on a battlefield or even at the scene of a ten-car pileup, a mobile blood warmer could come in handy.) The second didn't work out either. Billy did not give up. As always, he had another idea.

Every heart surgeon knew by the 1990s that the heart-lung machine had drawbacks. Stopping the heart during surgery was then and remains dangerous, and even patients who recover successfully from an operation can suffer serious side effects that have been attributed in studies to being "on the pump." (Temporary cognitive decline and personality changes are two side effects.)

But just as it was believed for centuries that no one could or should touch the heart, and later that attempting to operate on it was sure to cause certain death, it was believed as late as 1990 that performing surgery on a beating heart was impossible. "Like cutting a gemstone while you were on horseback," was the way one journalist put it. But Billy didn't see it that way. He was part of a new generation of surgeons who were trying to simplify operations that had become, maybe, just too complicated; the goal was to use advances in technology to create simpler and more successful operations. Billy wanted to bypass the bypass, as he put it. (The heart-lung machine, which allowed surgeons to circulate blood outside the actual heart and lungs during surgery, is not to be confused here with the coronary bypass operation, which allowed surgeons to literally circumvent blocked arteries by building new circulatory pathways out of veins taken from the legs, or man-made materials.)

Billy was not alone in his quest—many surgeons around the United States were thinking along the same lines. Like most good surgeons, he spent a lot of time traveling and talking with other doctors about recent advances in the field. On a visit to Johns Hopkins, Billy studied a technique developed by James Fonger, who had found a way to operate on beating hearts while holding them steady with something that looked like a two-pronged salad fork.

Back at Harvard, Billy tried it out, but found the heart still moved too much for his taste. Driving home from a long day in the OR in 1996, however, he had an inspiration. He pulled into his local Stop & Shop and roamed the aisles until he found the kitchen tools, and then started loading up on metal ladles, all sizes, the stronger the better.

Once in his basement in Brookline, Billy started pounding the ladles flat and adjusting the angles until he had one he liked. Then he cut a one-inch square right in the middle. Billy had a hunch that he could treat the heart like an egg in a basket by pressing the flattened ladle against the heart to hold it steady while he repaired the area visible through the window in the middle of the device.

Over the next few months, he tried his invention out on dogs and sheep, refining his design so that he was able to stabilize the beating heart to a greater and greater degree. Finally, in 1996, a patient gave his informed consent to let Billy skip the traditional heart-lung machine in favor of surgery with something that looked like a kitchen spatula. Fortunately for everyone, the operation was a success. The surgery went faster, and the patient made a faster recovery. There were more refinements—eventually Billy's creation looked like two spatulas held together with a retractor that clamped on the chest—and within the year, Billy Cohn had sold the Cohn Cardiac Stabilizer to Genzyme Surgical Products, one of the many medical device companies now ringing the Boston area as the field of bioengineering—building new body parts, in essence—was exploding. Billy would later describe his invention as having "all the complexity of a Happy Meal toy," but in the next few years it was put to use in sixty medical centers and more than 200,000 operations.

Along with his patent, Billy Cohn got a profile by Jerome Groopman in the *New Yorker* in 1999, with the headline "Heart Surgery, Unplugged." He was finally a rock star. So it was only natural that he would want to play with the coolest band in the world.

—⋀⋀—

Cooley had set up Surgical Associates of Texas in the early 1970s, a private practice of surgeons who maintained operating privileges at St. Luke's Hospital, the Texas Heart Institute's base of operations. He had not only perfected the coronary bypass operation by then, but was also thriving with his surgical assembly line. And if for some reason Cooley couldn't do the actual surgery, patients knew they were in good hands with one of his colleagues. That is, if anyone told them that had been the case.

This system made THI docs some of the richest in the world. A bypass operation cost around $60,000 back then, with most of it going to the surgeon. Being a member of the Texas Heart team at this time was the equivalent of getting a ticket punched at Harvard: it couldn't guarantee a hefty income for life, but it sure made it easier to get one.

At the top of the food chain, of course, was Cooley. He'd received the National Medal of Technology and Innovation from President Bill Clinton in 1998; he played golf with top-of-the-line Houstonians like former president George H. W. Bush and his secretary of state, James Baker. He was the old family friend George W. Bush turned to in 2000 to reassure himself that Dick Cheney was up to the rigors of campaigning as the Republican vice presidential nominee, despite his history of three heart attacks, bypass surgery, and two cardiac catheterizations. (Cooley was confident enough to give the OK without personally examining Cheney, who subsequently received an LVAD for his heart disease in 2010.) When the Denton Cooley Society held its annual meeting, they didn't go to the medical center's Marriott; they met instead in London, Hawaii, Puerto Rico, or Sun Valley. The meetings were underwritten by drug and device companies, and not just because Cooley himself was famously cheap—the companies wanted in too. The board of St. Luke's went to great lengths to make sure Cooley was happy: when a new medical office building opened across from the hospital, board members gave Cooley his own private apartment.

But just about everyone in Cooley's orbit became the medical equivalent of a master of the universe. Even someone like Bud

Frazier, whose income was (somewhat) limited by his commitment to research and an inability to care about getting really rich, still managed to indulge himself with rare books from a London dealer, and to save his beloved Anderson Fair music venue from extinction.

If you were a part of the THI team, you had the opportunity to indulge every whim, assuming you had time to do it. And of course, there were nurses and secretaries and all sorts of other attractive women who were more than willing to take a spin in whatever fancy car you chose to show off. Or join you for fancy dinners, or just meet you in one or another hospital call room. There were surgeons who indulged in ritalin and coke, and more. And there was the occasional hiccup: the wife of one of Cooley's associates shot and killed her husband in their River Oaks mansion, claiming he had abused her. She got off. "I don't know about you," Cooley joked to a colleague after visiting the scene on the day of the murder. "But I'm going home and hiding my guns."

But Cooley was getting older—in 2000, he was eighty and, like DeBakey, was never terribly interested in any succession plan. He continued operating until he was eighty-seven, and then turned to legacy building, traveling, lecturing, and working on an autobiography. But handing over the reins of his beloved Texas Heart Institute? Not on his to-do list. For a man on such intimate terms with the universality and unpredictability of death, Cooley was surprisingly difficult to engage on the subject of his own mortality.

It was left to St. Luke's CEO, a shrewd administrator by the name of Michael Jhin, to bring up the subject with Cooley. The two men had been a remarkable team for over a decade; they built St. Luke's into a five-star colossus. The Texas Heart Institute surgeons were, of course, the big draw. It was important to the doctors, the hospital, and even the city of Houston to keep THI's reputation glowing and St. Luke's income growing. But who would make sure that happened once Cooley stepped down?

On a flight to New York, relaxing in first class over drinks, Jhin brought up to Cooley the name of a young surgeon who was making quite a name for himself at Harvard. Of course, his skills in the operating room couldn't match Cooley's, but he had charisma kind of like Cooley's. He was a natural performer, and his enthusiasm was contagious, qualities that would be needed for attracting new donors and keeping old ones. And he was inventive too, an innovator, always ahead of the pack. And—drumroll, please—he was from Houston. He'd grown up here and graduated from Baylor College of Medicine, and he seemed anxious to come back. Maybe Cooley should take a look at this guy, Jhin suggested with all the care and delicacy of a soldier tiptoeing through a mine field.

Cooley nodded. He would think on it, he said.

—∿—

As it turned out, Billy Cohn was indeed anxious to get back to Houston. He was starting to feel that his only option was private practice—he had reached a dead end in Boston: "I did not just spend sixteen years to work with uninspiring guys, and I was really depressed." He was, after all, a heart surgery *innovator*, and the best place to do that was still the Texas Heart Institute. His idols in the medical field were Denton Cooley and Bud Frazier.

In the past, Billy had made a point of introducing himself to Bud at medical meetings and conferences. When he tells these stories, they have the rosy glow of hero worship, like Jimi Hendrix introducing himself to B. B. King. In each meeting—at least to hear Billy tell it—Bud remembers him a little more clearly than in the last, until finally, several years later, the bromance blossomed.

Bud is still fond of claiming that at a medical conference years ago, Billy told him that a pulseless/continuous-flow artificial heart would never work. To which he replied with his favorite punch line: "Well, I've got a calf down in the basement of the Texas Heart Institute that says otherwise."

It is a story that makes Billy wince. Yes, he had some questions, but they had to do with the lymphatic system and blood flow and a whole lot of technical stuff that most people have no interest in. "Am I the kind of guy who would say that any kind of technology wouldn't work?" he asked after being assigned the straight man role one time too many. "Bud takes great satisfaction in saying I knew it wouldn't work. *Of course* I knew it would work."

The interchange, repeated many times over the years, serves as a pretty good encapsulation of their relationship. That and the fact that Billy had no equal in building things and Bud understood the body with a savant-like sixth sense. They complemented each other; moreover, they needed each other in order to realize their ambitions.

As it turned out, Billy's designation of heir apparent had only been apparent to Michael Jhin. In fact, his invitation to join Texas Surgical Associates in 2004 did not even ensure that he was welcomed into the fold. There were already plenty of surgeons in the practice who were quite adept at performing heart surgery, and they made it clear they had no intention of making room for the hotshot from Harvard, even if he *was* from Houston. On a visit to Boston, Bud had warned Billy that he would have to cultivate his own group of cardiologists for referrals if he wanted to get in the operating room. But Billy didn't want to do that, because Billy wasn't interested in building a private practice.

He became like a racehorse put out to pasture. After two years at THI, in fact, it looked as though his career might be shifting in another direction: ABC asked Billy to audition for a new reality show called *Miracle Workers*, which, consciously or not, was developed to demonstrate that technology had made doctors the good guys again;

it was a small assist in the wake of ever-increasing medical costs and the fallout from managed care. The show was sort of a combination of *Queen for a Day*, *Marcus Welby, MD*, and the Discovery Channel.

A new kind of celebrity doctor was on the rise. If Cooley and De-Bakey were the stars of their generation, alternative medicine guru Andrew Weil, and Mehmet Oz, an esteemed cardiothoracic surgeon at Columbia University's Medical School, were turning themselves into brands. Both enjoyed the kind of multiplatform success—websites! books! products! Oprah!—that most day-to-day docs, warring with insurance companies and personal injury lawyers, could only dream of. (Oz did run into trouble when he endorsed diet pills that a Senate panel in 2014 deemed useless.)

But this was not to be Billy's future. The network canceled *Miracle Workers* after six episodes. The final show depicted an LVAD implanted by Billy and Bud on a woman whose cancer meds had destroyed her heart. Like the show, she didn't make it.

HEARTMATES

In 2003, a young man from El Salvador, with a thatch of lustrous dark hair that belied his weakened frame, came under Bud's care. He was dying of heart disease. THI was the last stop before he was forced to give in to his fate. The man's command of English was limited, and his family was not wealthy. He had worked as a car mechanic before he got sick.

But his timing was good. By that time, LVADs were losing their experimental reputation. A clinical trial of 129 patients with end-stage heart failure at Columbia University Medical School showed that the pumps reduced the risk of death by 48 percent, as compared with medication, and also substantially improved their quality of life. Bud groused about the trial at the time, claiming that it was unethical and unnecessary because everyone (i.e. him) already knew that the pumps worked better than meds.

Bud had been working with one of the device companies, Nimbus, on a new nonpulsatile implantable pump, which would eventually be called the HeartMate II. The pump was intended to be a great leap forward in heart assist devices: the HeartMate II was another axial flow pump, but it was much smaller. At an inch and a half long and weighing about twelve ounces—the size of Bud's thumb—it could fit in women, children, and smaller men. It was also designed with two speeds, one fixed and one called auto-speed, a kind of a manual transmission, whereby a patient could adjust the speed of the pump if he or she was feeling short of breath or was playing golf and needed a little boost.

The calf experiments went extremely well, and the FDA granted permission for human trials. That's when things began to go south: of the first ten patients, nine died. The one who lived did so because the surgeon took the pump out after two weeks. The FDA was about to put a stop to the trials when Bud and the team realized what was wrong: the manufacturer had used something called sintered titanium on the ends of the pump, a substance that roughed up the surface in pulsatile pumps, which made a safe place for clots to form on the membranes inside the device instead of clogging up the blood flow. But in a rapidly spinning pump the surface coating had the opposite effect: it grabbed bits of blood and gave it a place to settle, forming the clots that caused the fatal strokes in the early patients. The problem hadn't shown up in calves because calves had a higher blood pressure, which literally sucked blood through the pump, and covered up the problem. The solution seemed simple: to stop using sintered titanium. The FDA agreed to let the team try.

But there was another problem. By early 2000, Nimbus was nearly broke from its failed R&D. A couple of representatives flew to Houston to ask Bud to donate $600,000 to the company to keep going. But, as he told them, he was an academic surgeon. He was also helping to support his grown son Todd's career as a composer of operas—the Eastman School of Music and Juilliard graduate had created an opera about heart transplants called *Breath of Life*—and his daughter Allison's work as a writer and therapist. Both had spouses and children, and it was hard for Bud to deny them anything. "I make more than an English professor, but I don't have $600,000," he explained. In turn, they asked about Dr. Cooley. Would he contribute? "Remember Scrooge McDuck?" was Bud's response. If it hadn't been for another angel investor—the new head of a telecom company, who suffered from heart disease himself—the HeartMate II would have never come to be.

With the infusion of cash, Nimbus could afford to try again. Bud presented the option of experimental surgery to the dying young man from El Salvador, who agreed to take the chance. The operation went well. So well, in fact, that the man either didn't understand the nurse's instructions after his release from the hospital or didn't care. He didn't reappear for his follow-up appointment. In fact, he disappeared. Months went by with no sign of him. He literally vanished with $600,000 worth of experimental hardware in his chest.

It wasn't until a year later that he reappeared on Bud's doorstep, and that was only because he'd developed a small infection in the drive line of his device, a common problem with any sort of catheters, any medical apparatus that is exposed to the air.

What was a medical problem for the young man was something else entirely to Bud. He put his stethoscope to the patient's heart—and heard virtually nothing but the whooshing sound of the machine. The HeartMate II, which was supposed to keep the left ventricle going, had taken over almost all heart function. It was strong enough not just to push the blood out of the left ventricle into the body but to take up the work of the right side, getting blood into and out of the lungs as well. The machine had totally replaced his heart.

"Why didn't you come back?" a somewhat dazed Bud asked him.

The man shrugged. "I felt fine," he said.

It was then that Bud began to wonder—if a single HeartMate II worked that well, what would happen if someone could figure out how to put two HeartMate IIs together, one for the left side and one for the right, to make a permanent artificial heart?

That someone was Billy Cohn, working with Thoratec, which by this time had grown into one of the country's largest medical device companies. It boasted a team of engineers who had once worked on DeBakey's old LVAD—the one that was so close in design to the Jarvik 2000 but had been abandoned by its hedge fund backers.

Bud's simple-sounding idea would involve a pretty complex feat of biomedical engineering: a device designed to pump blood from the left side of the heart into the body would have to be redesigned to work with the right side, delivering blood to the lungs for oxygenation. The angles in the design of the HeartMate II would have to be changed to fit a different system, as would the pump speeds, to mimic a different rate of flow in a completely different part of the body. The right side of the heart was also more prone to clots; the lungs filtered them out only if they were small. Oddly enough, the right side of the heart also seemed to work better with some pulsing action. So the engineers had to figure out a way to build a faint pulse back into the HeartMate II.

With Thoratec's engineers engaged, Billy focused on a set of connectors to bridge one machine to the aorta and the other to the pulmonary system. He started shopping for parts, as always, at Home Depot, twisting cones out of various materials—silicone, rubber, drywall tape—until he had something that he thought might work.

The technical, legal, biological, governmental, financial, and, of course, interpersonal challenges were enormous, and five years passed in a heartbeat. By the mid-2000s, Billy and Bud had become the odd couple of THI, as different in their personalities as Jarvik and Wampler or DeBakey and Cooley. Billy was flamboyant, impulsive, and creative, someone who could envision a device in three dimensions long before it actually existed. Bud was erudite, thoughtful, and methodical; he could envision how a device would work in the body long before it was even built. The two men got on each other's nerves and sometimes bickered like a couple of brothers separated by just a few years.

Still, the partnership worked. Bud was then in his mid-sixties and continuing to put in endless days and nights in the operating room. (Staffers made grim jokes about "Bud time," because so many of his operations wound up taking place in the middle of the night. Bud was an easy touch when it came to interruptions.) Billy had a radically different sense of time—think speed of light versus glacial—and could put in more hours in the lab. Bud would have an idea—why not build in a septum, the central wall that separates the two sides of the heart?—and Billy would suggest reasons why that might not work, but then head home to his shop or the lab and start cobbling something together. Then the engineers would go to work, to come up with a working model. And Bud would razz Billy for being a doubter.

Billy and Bud tested iterations of this new double pump on more than forty calves. "We just did it and rigged 'em up," was the way Bud put it. The only one that died was a calf that got startled, reared back, and pulled out his drive lines from the console.

Money wasn't hard to come by. The Dunn Foundation, a fund supported by a Houston oil fortune, had long contributed to myriad enterprises in the Texas Medical Center. There was a Dunn Tower at Methodist Hospital, just for starters. Bud was well known to them, not just because of his international reputation but also because his best friend from the University of Texas was on the board. They pitched in half a million.

Their biggest problem, it turned out, was finding existing pumps to adapt and implant. At this point, the artificial heart business was going nowhere, while the LVAD business was rolling. At least five companies, along with Thoratec, were in the business in the United

States alone—Berlin Heart, Medtronics, and more—and European and Asian companies were also getting in on the act. The medical device business in general had exploded in the last decade or so, and the more complex the device, the more expensive. Heart assist devices sold for around $700,000 and Bud needed two for each calf implant. By 2009 or so, the HeartMate II was the bestselling LVAD on the market, keeping as many as twenty thousand patients alive. A continuous-flow pump, the only parts of the HeartMate II that lay outside the body were the small controller and the battery packs. Patients, according to the literature, could "once again enjoy their favorite activities, such as travel, golf, visiting family members, dancing, and playing an instrument."

Now Bud Frazier looked to be muddying the waters with another loony idea. Why should Thoratec devote time and money to an experimental total heart when the HeartMate II was already an enormous success, and the market for those needing total heart replacement was comparatively small? And, at $600,000 to $700,000 a pop, why should any medical device company hand over equipment for free, just to find out if two LVADs could work as well as a real heart?

So to get the parts they needed, Bud and Billy scavenged. In their earliest efforts to fuse two LVADs together, they used a Micromed pump—one of DeBakey's old pumps. As Bud put it, "there were a lot left over" when the company went under. They used some of Jarvik's pumps, but there weren't as many of those around, because Jarvik had never been able to get very many manufactured. Finally they managed to convince Thoratec to come up with the rest, either as a result of Bud's longtime association with the company or because he simply refused to go away.

By 2011, he was on the lookout for another end-of-life patient who was willing to take a chance on testing an experimental device, someone hovering in that fragile, twilit state closer to death than life.

Someone who had exhausted all other options, but who still hoped for one more chance to live.

That's when Craig Lewis appeared in the St. Luke's emergency room.

—⋀⋀—

When he wasn't in the OR, in the lab, needling Billy, or trying to relax while watching *The Wages of Fear* or the like on his office television, Bud tried to reconcile two pieces of another, more challenging puzzle: making peace between his mentors, Michael DeBakey and Denton Cooley. It was a widely held belief at the time that the competition between the two surgeons had actually helped to make the Texas Medical Center a global force in the treatment of heart disease. But the world of medicine had grown ever more specialized and ever more expensive in the span of their careers; the competition between the hospitals in the Texas Medical Center meant that after more than fifty years there were lots of pricey redundancies. Maybe a little collaboration going forward wouldn't be such a bad thing, especially since the enmity between the Cooley forces and the DeBakey loyalists included not just heart surgeons but the lowest tech, who probably hadn't been born when the fight started.

Besides that, Bud knew that Cooley was bothered that his own chief still treated him like a pariah. As he moved into his eighties, Cooley spoke more and more often of wanting to make amends; he didn't want to apologize, exactly—Cooley never stopped believing DeBakey would never have implanted Liotta's heart in a human patient—but he did want to thank DeBakey for bringing him to Houston and inspiring him to launch all that followed. As for De-Bakey, he continued to insist, as did his sisters and at least one son, that there had never been a feud. It was Team DeBakey's way of saying that Denton Cooley had simply ceased to exist. Like a Soviet traitor in the old Politburo, he had been excised from their collective memory.

As of 2004, building an artificial heart from scratch looked like an easier job than making peace between two old and very proud men. That was the year Bud organized a conference on the history of the LVAD at the Texas Heart Institute and invited DeBakey to come. To the astonishment of virtually everyone involved, he accepted, showing up in a wheelchair and, at ninety-six, giving a lucid, engaging talk on his early work with heart pumps from a podium with the Texas Heart Institute logo.

Cooley was there too. He listened attentively but did not go near the stage. DeBakey made no acknowledgment of Cooley either; he gave his talk and left the auditorium immediately.

A year or so later, Cooley nearly lost any chance for reconciliation. DeBakey nearly died of a dissecting aortic aneurysm, which meant that the inner lining of his aorta was falling apart, like old cloth. DeBakey diagnosed his condition alone while in his study. As the *New York Times* would point out a few months later, no one was more qualified to make that diagnosis; DeBakey had devised the artificial graft used in the delicate surgery that was subsequently applied around the world to repair torn aortas.

Not surprisingly, the prospect of performing that surgery on DeBakey himself turned many of his protégés into ninnies. Nobody wanted to be remembered as the surgeon who lost Michael DeBakey on the operating table. After all, he had a wife, their thirty-one-year-old daughter, two grown sons from his first marriage, and two elderly sisters who remained financially and emotionally dependent on him. Much more terrifying was the fact that he was Michael DeBakey, who had built Baylor College of Medicine and Methodist

Hospital and changed the face of national and global health. Operating on him without success was a surefire career-killer.

The risks were enormous: no one in their nineties is an ideal candidate for major surgery. In fact, DeBakey had written sensible instructions years before requesting that no extreme measures be taken to save his life.

DeBakey's wife, however, was not ready to let go. Proving herself as relentless as her husband, Katrin browbeat Methodist Hospital's ethics committee into approving the operation when its members were dragging their heels, petrified of making the wrong decision.

After a great deal of soul-searching, DeBakey's longtime associate George Noon agreed to perform the repair. The seven-hour operation included the use of an updated Dacron graft similar to the one DeBakey had perfected so many decades before, in the 1950s. DeBakey spent several rocky months recovering in his hospital's ICU, but by the end of 2006, he was back at home in his white brick mansion on Cherokee and soon after was once again speeding through Methodist's corridors on an electric scooter.

—⌇—

DeBakey's near-death experience resonated deeply with Cooley. Driving home from his THI office on a crisp day in January 2007, he turned on impulse onto DeBakey's street and parked his car. For one of the few times in his life, he was ambivalent. Eventually he got out of his car, stepped to the front door, and rang the bell, and when a startled Katrin answered, he asked to speak with DeBakey. She kept him cooling his heels in the living room for about twenty minutes and then came back to declare that DeBakey was asleep.

"Why don't you write him a note?" Bud suggested when Cooley told him what had happened. So he did, asking to visit in order to thank DeBakey for the influence he'd had on Cooley's life and career. "Especially, I am grateful for the opportunity you provided me more than 50 years ago to become established at Baylor and to be inspired by your work ethic and ambition," he wrote. Cooley asked to pay a call at DeBakey's convenience. He never got an answer.

Finally George Noon and Bud Frazier stepped in and came up with a scheme. By that time, there had been plenty of fallout from the forty-year-old feud, including the existence of not one but *two* organizations for honoring the surgeons' trainees: the Denton Cooley Cardiovascular Surgical Society and the Michael E. DeBakey International Surgical Society. Maybe, the doctors posited, it was time for the Cooley Society to give DeBakey an award for his achievements and throw in an honorary membership. It was the rare superstar surgeon who could turn down a big award, especially from a competitor.

And sure enough, on October 27, 2007, DeBakey drove his motorized wheelchair into the THI auditorium in the sunlit Denton A. Cooley wing to accept the honor. This time Cooley did speak to DeBakey, and DeBakey said he would treasure the award and find a place for it in his library. Ostensibly he meant the one he was then building at Baylor to house his papers and inventions, including various heart pumps, a replica of the sewing machine upon which he had made the Dacron graft, and an actual-sized reproduction of DeBakey's operating room from the 1960s.

More reconciliations would follow. DeBakey invited Cooley to the ceremony in which he received the Congressional Gold Medal from President George W. Bush in April 2008. (Cooley, a multimillionaire, opted to share a hotel room with Bud.) And then, a month later, the DeBakey International Surgical Society gave Cooley a lifetime achievement award and honorary membership.

The most meaningful rapprochement, however, probably took

place away from the public eye. DeBakey had expressed an interest in watching one of the implants Bud and Billy had been working on with the tandem artificial heart. In December 2007, Bud invited him to the operating room in the animal lab, when they were trying an experiment with two of DeBakey's old Micromed pumps.

He agreed to come, as did Cooley. It was the first time the two had been in an operating room together in decades, even though this one was used for animals. Cooley walked in under his own power; DeBakey was in his wheelchair, and someone draped him in a paper surgical gown and mask. The two men positioned themselves in the back, chatting quietly and amiably, watching on one of the monitors as Bud worked. They were like retired quarterbacks evaluating a game that was just the same and yet completely different from the one they had played for so long.

DeBakey died in July 2008, just a few months shy of his 100th birthday. Thousands came to a viewing when, at the request of Katrin, he lay in state at Houston's City Hall—the first time the building was put to that use in its seventy-year history. In his coffin, DeBakey was dressed in his white coat and royal-blue scrubs, along with a cloth surgical cap and a mask pulled down under his chin.

Riding back from the event with Bud, Cooley was pensive. He told Bud he wanted his funeral in his childhood church on Main Street. He said he'd be just fine in a blue serge suit. "I don't want anything elaborate," he said.

—⌁—

"You can operate on really sick people but everything has to go right," DeBakey told Bud many years ago. The warning came back to Bud in March 2011 as he prepared Craig Lewis for surgery.

Bud had followed all the FDA procedures for emergency use: in the space of about 48 hours, Bud and Billy's team filled out countless federal forms, and more for the HeartMate II's manufacturer. They had won permission from the hospital to proceed with the operation, though that had turned out to be more difficult than Bud had anticipated. The review board was wary: lawsuits, sanctions—any number of things could go wrong if the operation went bad, which it was likely to do. One administrator pointed out the obvious: the doctors hadn't even done one implantation in a person, which was, of course, the point. With Craig Lewis' chances diminishing by the second, however, the hospital administration finally agreed to let Bud proceed.

So on a sunny spring day in 2011, when a lot of Houstonians were enjoying blooming azaleas and sweet Gulf breezes, Bud stood in the Texas Heart Institute's largest operating room. Unlike virtually everyone else circling around him, he was calm. He figured the two HeartMate IIs would work in Lewis' chest at least as well as they had worked in the calves. He had been here many times before, or at least that's what he told himself.

A heart-lung machine had already taken over for Lewis' ailing heart. He was draped from head to toe, except for a chasm where an associate had opened up his chest, so that his diseased heart sat exposed, barely beating, the color of rotting meat. There were so many tubes and wires coming in and out of his body that a less experienced surgeon might have been terrified of tripping, but Cohn and Frazier moved about effortlessly and economically, never quite standing up to their full height as they focused on the patient on the table. Billy, as usual, was responsible for cracking the jokes. Bud chuckled whether he found them funny or not.

He began by cutting out virtually all of Lewis' diseased heart. His hands, encased in yellow gloves, grew redder with blood by the minute as he snipped away at the arteries and veins holding Lewis' heart in place, until finally he lifted the diseased organ out of Lewis' chest, casually handing it to a nurse, who unceremoniously put it in a cooler for pathology. And then Frazier and Cohn began stitching their artificial heart into Craig Lewis' body, a process that would take about nine hours. Frazier could feel the crowd of doctors and nurses leaning into the skylight in the viewing area above him. But he never looked up, not once.

—⋀⋀—

Relatives of patients are not allowed to watch operations, so the first glimpse Linda Lewis got of her husband was the next morning when she entered his hospital room. He was sitting up in bed, surrounded by monitors, tapping away on his computer.

One of the doctors examining Craig beckoned her closer. "Want to hear it?" he asked, guiding her toward the bed. Linda leaned in and put her ear to Craig's chest and waited. Then she shifted her body, so that she could press just a little harder. There was almost nothing to hear. No *thump-thump*; just a faint whirring somewhere way down deep inside. She was hearing the sound of the first non-pulsatile artificial heart ever put inside a human.

Over the next few weeks, Craig Lewis once again became the person he'd been before the illness began to claim him. He greeted Linda with a broad smile and a wave. He asked for ice cream. He worked on his laptop. He graciously accepted a visit from Cooley and other heart surgeons from around the medical center, who entered his room stunned to see what Bud and Billy had done.

But amyloidosis is fatal, and the disease continued its steady, devastating march through Lewis' body, picking off his organs one by one. Five weeks after the surgery, he was gone. Linda's only consolation was that her husband's death would have value going forward. "If it didn't help Craig, it would help somebody down the line," she told Bud.

Before she took her husband's body home for burial, a pathologist removed his man-made heart. Bud ran some tests on the mechanics, and it continued to work well, spinning and whirring cheerily like a kid's toy. It might still have been working in Lewis if not for the amyloidosis. The patient died, but in many ways the operation was a success.

THE AUSTRALIAN GUY

When pressed for time, Billy Cohn lapsed into irritability, and he was often pressed for time due to the chaotic nature of his surgical career and the persistent urgency of his own internal state. This may have been why, in September 2011, he was annoyed that his secretary had put a name on his calendar he did not recognize. Who the hell was Daniel Timms?

Billy was working on all sorts of things at the time, including a safer, easier device for catheterizing dialysis patients, and improvements to the twin turbine artificial heart that had gone into Craig Lewis. He and Bud had also more quietly put that same device in a dying woman, after her husband begged them to give it a try. Really, it was far too late for such a procedure—Bud was always one for a Hail Mary pass—and she died on the operating table.

Still, the attendant publicity of the first operation had made Cohn, along with Frazier, a celebrity in worlds far beyond their fields of expertise—they were a media hit on everything from CNN to Al Jazeera, which featured an X-ray of Lewis' artificial heart looking like a set of Siamese-twin spark plugs in his chest. Billy and Bud gave a TEDMED talk, which was the 2012 equivalent to getting on the cover of *Life* magazine.

Billy was inclined to think of all publicity as good publicity—he loved being a star, so there wasn't much downside. But, since Lewis, his office had been flooded with calls from other self-described medical innovators. Someone wanted to show him a special device that would power the heart through a fitting in a shoe, for instance. Then there was the guy with the power source that he promised mysteriously floated in a giant rotating sphere. Billy offered his opinion to as many inventors as patiently as he could, but sometimes he listened while rearranging papers and gadgets on his desk and checking his email and his texts.

He had not expected the meeting with this Timms character to go any differently. "Another crackpot with a backpack full of crap," was the way he put it to himself. Yes, a brief meeting with Bud and another colleague was slowly emerging from his memory—something about an Australian guy who was doing some interesting things in the field of rotary pumps. Maybe this guy had an answer to some problems they'd been having with blood clots in their own pumps. Sure, Billy thought. Whatever. Maybe Timms' ideas would be cool, maybe they would be goofy.

Timms himself *was* goofy, though he probably seemed less so to the likes of Billy and Bud. He was a man who was otherwise engaged: Timms came into Billy's office looking like someone who hadn't slept in months—because he hadn't—his hazel eyes red-rimmed, his jeans torn, his shirt untucked, and his stubble much closer to an eight o'clock shadow than a five o'clock.

The guy wasn't much on pleasantries. Timms started taking things out of his scuffed, soiled, seemingly bottomless backpack—notebook, laptop, red and blue connector tubes, et cetera—and placing them on Billy's desk. Unlike many people, he seemed unafraid that he might be swallowed by the Billysphere. Timms was chattering in an Aussie accent about two cars with two engines linked together on the same highway, trying to make some kind of point.

Finally Timms pulled out something wrapped in an old T-shirt. It looked like it had been made by a hobbyist during the midcentury modern period but was in fact a model for a new kind of artificial heart: a small plastic cylinder, about three inches in diameter, with stubby protrusions. Timms put his hands to either side of the prototype and twisted it along a seam, opening it like a jar of shoe polish. Inside was something new and different: unlike so many of the heart pumps Billy had seen, this one was centrifugal, round instead of long and narrow.

To explain how it would work, Timms popped open his laptop and showed Cohn an animated film. It was pretty simple: Inside was a rotor that was suspended courtesy of an invisible but powerful magnetic field. Magnets, reminiscent of the bearings suspended in Wampler's and Jarvik's design, directed the spinning of the rotor, which was two-sided; it could simultaneously spin blood in two directions, to the body and the lungs. There was no pump, so there was no pulse, though one could be built in if necessary. It seemed to work as simply as two lanes of the same superhighway. Well, thought Cohn, lots of things work perfectly in animation that don't work so hot in real life.

Timms continued to talk at a speedy clip, as if he was afraid Cohn would start rearranging the doodads on his desk at any minute. This artificial heart had a lot of advantages that other devices currently in development did not. Most important, it could automatically adjust blood flow to a person's needs.

This promise stopped Billy cold. If Timms was right, he had managed to do something that had never been done before. Ever. A normal heart pumps according to the body's physical needs. That is, when you get up from a chair, or dash up a flight of stairs, the heart pumps harder to keep the blood flowing, according to what is known as the Frank-Starling Law. The same thing happens if you get up too fast after a nap—you get dizzy—or sit too long with one leg tucked under. The heart knows that some part of the body needs more flow, and gets it done. No artificial heart had ever come close to doing anything like that.

Billy, who had a tendency to slump back in his chair and wiggle one foot when he was only mildly interested, was now sitting up straight and actually listening. The heart that he and Bud had put in Craig Lewis flowed at a constant rate. Some changes could be made with manual controls with the HeartMate II, but they'd never been able to come up with a pump that could automatically adjust blood flow to the body's needs. In fact, clots had killed several calves in their experiments and probably would have killed Lewis if he had lived long enough. Now here was this kid—who was not even an MD, much less a heart surgeon—who appeared to have solved the problem.

This is crazy, Billy told himself. But the more Timms talked—he didn't really need to draw much breath to continue—the more Billy began to suspect that Daniel Timms was the farthest thing from a crackpot there was.

Billy had a gift for knowing whether something was workable or not. He also knew enough about artificial heart technology to be able to see the device's other advantages (though Timms went on to enumerate them). This heart was smaller than any other artificial heart he'd ever seen—that meant it could be implanted in women and children, not just oversized men, who made up the vast majority of patients willing to try such devices in the past. Also—and this was important—Timms' heart, with just one moving part, was a lot less fragile. Craig Lewis' device had more than fifty moving parts, any of which could break at any time, causing a life-threatening disaster. Imagine, for instance, a car that had only one moving part under the hood. It was that revolutionary.

And this heart could go and go; designed so that no part touched the sides, there was far less opportunity for wear and tear. Timms figured his machine should last five to ten years. Yes, one drawback was that it was currently powered outside the body with a battery pack, but so was every other heart assist device. Timms, however, was already working on plans to implant the entire system inside the body; a patient would eventually be able to regulate himself just by pressing a button under his skin.

Billy stared down at the metal cylinder Daniel was now balancing lovingly in his hands. It was, he knew, the most highly evolved artificial heart he had ever seen.

"How have you done this?" he asked Daniel.

"It's just something I came up with," Daniel answered, but he had an expression Billy knew all too well: the face of a magician who'd pulled off a seemingly impossible trick.

—∿—

Daniel Timms carries on his iPhone a photo of a photo, something his mother sent him while he was working far away from home. The picture, which dates to the 1980s, is washed-out, the tropical color of Daniel's house in the Brisbane suburb of Ferny Hills faded by the years. Still, it's a pretty archetypal scene, a boy and his father working on a backyard project. The boy, Daniel, is about eight, wispy and blond; his father, Gary, is all sinew and muscle, with a thick beard and a halo of brown curls around his head. They appear to be building a world in miniature—rock walls and waterfalls, mountain peaks eroded by swirling rivers—and something about their postures, the boy's eager, the father's calm, tells you a lot about where Daniel came from, literally and psychically.

Like Denton Cooley and Billy Cohn, Timms spent an inordinate amount of time building things in his youth—his father was a plumber by trade, but also something of a mechanical savant who never got the opportunity to go to college. Daniel didn't grow up wealthy—in that regard he has more in common with Frazier than Cooley or Cohn—but his closeness with his father would always set him apart. He was coached in the most affectionate way to carry the family banner forward toward some form of a better life. Daniel's mother, Karen, was a high school science teacher and welcomed Daniel to her lab before and after school to check out other students' projects.

So at an early age Daniel became not just a devotee of scientific inquiry but something of a prodigy when it came to gravity and flow, circulation and currents. His parents saved money for college, and Daniel was headed to Queensland University of Technology with plans to become an engineer. He might have grown up to be another successful Brisbane engineer, spending weekends building mountains and channeling rivers with his own son while his father looked on.

Instead, what happened next was the sort of dramatic event that makes for (and eventually did become) manna to newspaper feature writers. Gary Timms had a massive heart attack at fifty-five, collapsing at home on a weekday afternoon while the sun was shining and the palm trees outside swayed obliviously in the breeze. His life would never be quite the same after that, and neither would Daniel's.

To be close to a parent who is severely ill is an exercise in helplessness and delusion. Gary Timms' world constricted: he had little energy for his job, and soon had to stop working. The flesh hung on his once muscular frame, and his face, once brown from the Australian sun, turned ashen. There are grown sons with sick fathers who would content themselves with calling more often or committing to more frequent Sunday visits, but Daniel had other ideas. By 2001, he was twenty-two and working on his PhD, the subject of which, not surprisingly, was heart disease. The field of bioengineering was then exploding. No longer was a bioengineer just an engineer who happened to work with doctors; now a specialist in bioengineering was a new kind of expert who could apply the computer modeling once used to build bridges or skyscrapers to the needs of the body, estimating the reaction of any kind of biological or physiological system to a change in its environment. Modern-day ventilators, pacemakers, and respirators had been updated using this technology, and the implantation of an artificial hip or knee joint, miraculous in the 1980s, was routine by the time Daniel Timms was a young adult.

To Daniel and his father, then, it seemed perfectly natural that they would start working on a mechanical replacement for a diseased heart. In his room one day, Daniel sat down and sketched a device that drew on his extensive knowledge of physics and plumbing. The human body was, to him, just another engineering system; you could make a water pump for a mine, or a blood pump for humans. But if you only focused on one part of a system or a body, you could miss the solution you were seeking. A pump—or the heart—was always part of a larger system. Daniel started drawing, and when he finished his own heart was pounding. "Fuck yeah," he wrote under the sketch.

Thus began one of the more unlikely but not entirely out of the ordinary journeys in modern medicine. It was not long before the shed in the Timms backyard overflowed with molds and models—resembling a tidier, less manic version of Billy Cohn's man-cave garage in Houston, but a less pristine environment than Robert Jarvik's. Pressed for space, father and son eventually moved their lathe into the kitchen and, literally, started cooking projects in the family oven. Making slow but steady progress, they then set up a satellite office in the plumbing section of Bunnings, the Brisbane equivalent of Home Depot. In the beginning, they told the truth when passersby noticed the labyrinth of pipes Timms and his father set out on the floor. "We're trying to build a replica of the body's circulatory system to help us create an artificial heart," one of them would explain, looking up from the maze on the floor. But then word spread, and they started drawing a crowd. "We're building a fish tank," they started saying.

It was so much better to believe you could solve a problem, or cure a disease, than to sit by helplessly and watch a parent deteriorate. When Daniel wasn't refining his design, he was reading everything he could about artificial hearts, working as tirelessly as a scholarship student determined to be number one in his fancy prep school. He read about Cooley's ill-fated implantation of Liotta's heart, and studied the case of Barney Clark. He immersed himself in the development of left ventricular assist devices, the history of Rich Wampler and his Hemopump.

The world of artificial heart enthusiasts is very small, and it wasn't long before Daniel was carrying a mental Rolodex of who was doing what around the world. There were people working on artificial hearts out in Tucson, where SynCardia, the company that was previously Jarvik's Symbion, was making a name for itself with what they called a Total Artificial Heart. The company was doing well: FDA trials were in effect (in 2004, the device was approved as a bridge to transplant), and there were high hopes it could be used as a permanent replacement eventually. But to Frazier and Cohn—and Timms—the SynCardia device was, essentially, the latest iteration of the Jarvik-7 with a power console that could now be carried in a shoulder bag. The company was also working on a smaller version for women and children—Bud Frazier would implant them. But to continuous-flow believers, it was still an old-fashioned pulsatile pump with the same old attendant problems, durability being the most obvious.

A French company called Carmat had also been working on an artificial heart, but it was a complex device, also pulsatile, with myriad moving parts and a completion schedule that remained cloudy. Then there was the great cardiac powerhouse that was the Cleveland Clinic. Supposedly, researchers there were working on an artificial heart, but no one seemed to know much about it. Rich Wampler, too, was working on something in Oregon.

The name that came up most often when Daniel researched the literature was that of Dr. O. H. Frazier in Houston, Texas—he seemed to be the only heart surgeon who believed, like Daniel, that continuous flow was the way to go and that a pulse was something a person with an artificial heart could do without. If Daniel read five hundred papers on the pulseless heart, one hundred of them would be written by the Texas surgeon.

Daniel had never been out of Australia before, but now he began to use his small savings to track down some of the people he read about. In 2001, he took his first trip away from home, heading to Tokyo, where he had already Skyped with a young expert, Nobuyuki Kurita, who was doing unique work in magnetic levitation. Fortunately, Kurita spoke English, the two hit it off, and Kurita was willing to accept the trade Daniel proposed: his expertise in mechanical engineering for Kurita's expertise in creating a magnetic suspension system. Japanese trains had been running on such a system, called maglev, for at least a decade. Why couldn't you put one in the body? After all, Wampler and Jarvik had already used magnetic bearings to keep axial pumps turning. Daniel's design would just replace the bearings with more powerful, computer-directed magnets that would allow his device to be suspended—fewer parts and less wear.

From Japan Daniel went to Germany, where he spent nearly two years, off and on, studying pumps. And then to Sweden. There were trips to Athens and Egypt to track down particular experts in everything from software design to rotor heights and widths. There were no nights in five-star hotels or meals in fancy restaurants. Not only was he broke, but he had no interest in the high life. Daniel slept on couches and bartered his expertise for some tiny piece of information that might help advance his cause. Somehow, Daniel stretched his small funds to get to lectures around the globe, where he usually sat in the back, ever silent. When he heard Dr. Frazier would be speaking, Daniel stalked him like a bounty hunter, in packed lecture halls, never daring to introduce himself, but always thinking, "One day I will have something to show you."

—〰—

The invention of a pulseless heart might have seemed radical but plausible to people on the cutting edge of biomedical engineering, but back home in Brisbane Timms was not getting much support. He was twenty-two when he took his device to a group at the Prince Charles Hospital in Brisbane, in 2001. It isn't hard to envision the response of a group of heart surgeons corralled around a conference table while being asked to consider the work of an unknown engineer. One surgeon, after hearing Daniel's pitch, started pounding on the table like an angry diplomat in a United Nations debate: No artificial heart could ever be made to work without a pulse. Not ever. And who was Daniel to think otherwise?

Meanwhile, Gary Timms was slipping away. In 2004, he needed more surgery, this time to replace a leaking heart valve. He did not improve. The backyard landscapes and the experiments at Bunnings seemed long, long ago. Daniel quickened his pace, living to the beat of an accelerating internal stopwatch. He went without sleep, forgot to eat, took so many planes to so many places that at times he forgot, briefly, where he was and why he had come. He was twenty-seven when his father died in 2006. After the funeral, he hit the road again.

Daniel had the true obsessive's immunity to rejection. Plenty of people told him how and why his device wouldn't work—most frequently because no one believed you could have an artificial heart that didn't also have a pulse. But what he told himself was this: no one ever said stop. That sliver of encouragement was enough. Eventually Daniel befriended a critical care expert at Prince Charles Hospital in Brisbane, a baby-faced, good-natured soul named John Fraser who, if he didn't understand exactly what Daniel was doing, sensed that the sleepless wraith whom he often heard banging on metal objects in an adjacent office was doing something of value.

He used his influence to get Daniel a job and a lab in the clinical science department, and threw in a new couch covered in black vinyl. It took a very short time for the couch to take on Daniel's rumpled, weary mien.

Over the next three years, he did not allow himself to doubt. He had no idea, really, whether the device would work, which was admittedly a drawback in what was becoming a constant scramble for cash. The investors he met saw the need for a new approach, but they also wanted a sure thing.

The only sure thing Daniel had to show for those long, hard years was his team. Most of them were young men in their twenties. Drawn from all over the world, they were not always so well versed in English, but they were completely conversant with what Daniel was trying to do. To a one, they fell in line Pied Piper style, connecting via text, email, and Skype, holding up drawings and parts and graphs on the computer screen, making adjustments with clicks of their keyboards. Finally they were ready for short-term animal testing. They tried first in Australia, and then again in Taiwan. Both animals died on the operating table.

The fact that Daniel had been publishing papers on his work during this time, however, had helped him move from a twentysomething tyro to a thirtysomething colleague in the world of pulseless heart assist devices. Instead of sitting in the backs of auditoriums, he was now invited to talk about his work to small, ever more prestigious groups. In fact, the International Society for Heart and Lung Transplantation invited Daniel to come to Paris in April 2009. He realized he would need a suit and a shave.

Daniel was not a natural speaker. He knew exactly what was at stake, but he had an engineer's emotive range, especially in public, and especially before a group as important as this, a global organization with over three thousand members—surgeons, nurses, anesthesiologists, pulmonologists, and so on, medical professionals who had dedicated their lives to eradicating heart and lung diseases. He practiced his presentation over and over again, hoping to appear relaxed and accessible. Still, on the podium, Daniel fell back on old habits and read his speech to the crowd. He was so afraid of making a mistake that he didn't notice one person in the audience listening intently: O. H. Frazier.

At the end of Daniel's talk, Bud got slowly to his feet and turned to address the crowd. "This," he said, "is going to be the future of total artificial hearts." Daniel was so shocked that he waited too long to find Frazier and introduce himself after his speech—Bud was already gone.

Then, at a Singapore conference in 2011, he met a man named Steve Parnis, who was about Daniel's age but balding and far more gregarious. Parnis, it turned out, was from the Texas Heart Institute and had been following Daniel's work with interest. Daniel would also soon learn that Parnis was part of Frazier's seat-of-the-pants operation. Bud carried on the tradition of DeBakey and Cooley, hiring expert oddballs—or oddball experts—who didn't necessarily have documentation for their expertise. After Dr. Norman's departure, Bud upgraded by hiring trained veterinarians to work 24/7. Over time, the place began to resemble the snazziest animal ICU, with the pigs and calves getting better care than a lot of humans who couldn't get into St. Luke's. Bud also partnered with a Croatian immigrant named Branislav Radovancevic, known as Brano, a much beloved researcher who never managed to get his US medical degree. And then there was Parnis. He wasn't an MD or a veterinarian, but by that time had been performing operations on animals for more than twenty years in the THI lab under Bud's direction. As such, Parnis was pretty up to speed on artificial hearts.

He and Daniel talked about continuous flow for at least an hour; from a distance, they could have been mistaken for two guys obsessing about craft beers or Super Bowl contenders. In parting, Parnis offered the Texans' typical farewell: if Daniel ever made it to Houston, he'd be happy to show him around. Who knew? Maybe he had something to teach Frazier and Cohn.

As it turned out, Daniel *was* going to be in the United States in a few months, at a conference in Louisville. He'd love to stop by, Daniel said casually, never letting Parnis know how desperate he was to get to Houston.

MATILDA

Billy Cohn was good at a lot of things, but one of the things he was very good at was raising money. "Show me a homeless guy and I'll get five bucks out of him," he liked to say, which may not have been politically correct but was reflective of the source. At this particular time—the spring of 2012—he couldn't get Daniel Timms and his device out of his mind.

There were not very many people who understood, intuitively and intellectually, what Daniel had done, but Billy was one of them. He realized that Daniel Timms had come up with something so much better than anything Billy himself could have ever invented, even though Billy had come up with a design for a magnetically powered artificial heart several years earlier and still had the file on his laptop. But here was the thing: Daniel had *actually made one*. As inspired as Billy was, he was not an engineer. And Daniel was a generation younger, which meant that he had been able to ride a wave of technological innovation to an answer: advances in magnetic levitation were part of it, but also the simplest, most obvious things like Skype, which had allowed a diverse team of experts to work together even when they were thousands of miles apart.

In other words, Billy Cohn, no stranger to genius himself, was pretty sure that Daniel Timms' device had solved many of the problems that had held Bud and him back with their twin HeartMate IIs. Daniel—with the help of the medical team at the Texas Heart Institute, of course—could be on his way to inventing the first true artificial heart.

After their first meeting in early 2012, Daniel became like a magpie building a high-tech nest, flying off to Taiwan or Brisbane or God knows where to pick up a paying engineering gig and/or a little more knowledge, and then circling back to THI to put this newest discovery to use. Oblivious to the intense interest of the women hovering around him—the nurses, the techs, the receptionists, all of whom were standing at the ready to provide relief from his labors—Daniel did what he had always done, which was to work around the clock in his singular, solitary role as keeper of the Bivacor, the name of the device he had created.

No one in their right mind would describe Daniel as flexible, but he was slowly learning the THI way, which, when it came to experimentation, was still governed by the old THI ethos of try first and then figure out what went wrong and how to fix it. Daniel's first lesson occurred in the early summer of 2012, on a hot June day with temperatures he would probably have been oblivious to. He had flown into Houston with his usual encumbrances—the Bivacor in his backpack and not much else—and started to get ready for another of what had become a series of implantations in calves. All of the experiments to this date had been of the "acute" variety, which in medical research argot meant that the animals were short-termers: the scientists tried one thing or another but the animal never woke up from its drug-induced slumber. In this case, a calf would be allowed to live under observation long enough to confirm the success or failure of some new modification—some refinement of the Bivacor—that is, if they could wake the animal at all. In med language, this would be a "chronic" experiment because the animal got a stay of execution.

In those days, Daniel did all the prep work himself—making sure the device was ready to go, along with the software program that ran it—because there wasn't any money to bring in any of his far-flung team members to help him run an experiment. This situation proved particularly inconvenient when Steve Parnis sauntered into the lab and asked what time tomorrow Daniel would have the Bivacor ready.

"What are you talking about?" Daniel asked. He was sitting on a metal stool, surrounded by coils and casts and machine parts of indeterminate use to a layperson. "I've got, like, five days."

When it came to THI work habits, no one ever put much of a premium on communication—especially communicating about scheduling, because schedules changed so often. Parnis was one of those poor souls charged with making order out of chaos. "No," he explained, "you've got to have it ready tomorrow so we can sterilize it."

Unlike the old days, there are now many regulations controlling the ethical treatment of lab animals, some dictated by the US government via the FDA, and some THI's own. One of them is that you don't put a nonsterile device in an animal you intend to wake up—a chronic case—because otherwise you might be sentencing the animal to a painful, deadly infection. This information was familiar to Daniel in a general way, but he hadn't reached that specific crossroads as yet.

"Sterilize it for what?" Daniel asked, which was a perfectly legitimate question, because he had been thinking that, like all previous experiments, this one was to be acute. But here was Steve, talking like a reasonable person but using words that changed the game entirely.

"We can't put it in the animal unsterile if we're going to wake up the animal," he said slowly, as if he were talking to a child.

"Wake up the animal? What are you talking about?" Daniel asked. When he was alarmed, his speech picked up speed. It was doing that now.

It seemed that Billy and Bud had decided they should try to wake up the calf. Why not? They'd learn a lot more a lot sooner.

At times like these, Daniel revealed a nimbleness that was not always so apparent. In other words, he knew there was no point in arguing. "How long have I got?" he asked, in the tone of a condemned man. It usually took him about five days to prepare for an implantation.

A day and a half or so, Steve told him.

The next thirty-six hours were, for Daniel, a period of frantic activity followed by excruciating separation anxiety. He had always been able to keep the Bivacor device within easy reach, and now it had been whisked away, into some sterilizer, all alone. Daniel could think of nothing to do with himself with the free time. He didn't, for instance, visit any Houston tourist sites, like the slowly moldering Astrodome, aka the Eighth Wonder of the World, or the enormous port that included the Houston Ship Channel. The world-famous art at the Menil Collection or a performance by the Houston Grand Opera did not come to mind, nor did it occur to him to strike out for one of Houston's infamous "men's clubs," souped-up strip joints that were designed to imitate fancy frat houses or nineteenth-century English smoking rooms. He couldn't even take in a movie or go out for a burger. All he could think about was, "What if it doesn't work?"

That terror lingered and deepened on the morning he found himself in front of his computer console in the lab's operating room, wearing blue scrubs and a mask over his face, so that only his bloodshot blue eyes were showing.

There was a crush as word had spread about the upcoming implantation. People in scrubs already had their cellphone cameras at the ready, flouting all sorts of security rules. The light over the operating table was almost blinding, and brought a little heat to a room that felt like a sub-zero day in Juneau. A TV monitor was already focused on the patient, virtually invisible beneath a sky-blue drape except for the brown hoofs that stuck out from the large bovine body on the operating table like small piers awaiting the crest of a gigantic wave. The calf had no name, because in the world of animal research, it was considered bad luck to name an animal before she survived an operation. She was good-sized, about 130 pounds, and lying on her side. The entrance to her heart lay open like a crater, its circumference ringed with the garish yellow of Betadine antiseptic solution. Parnis had come in earlier and opened the chest, and now he was preparing to remove the heart and connect the calf's major arteries to the heart-lung machine that would keep her alive until, they hoped, the implanted Bivacor could take over.

After about an hour, a tech arrived in blue scrubs and a paper gown, her face obscured by a mask and the obligatory, universally unflattering paper cap. She was carrying a metal bowl filled with sterile solution in which the Bivacor floated, as if it were an offering, or, maybe, the $40 entrée at one of Houston's most exclusive restaurants. That is, if an entrée looked like a small metal cylinder with a few curved protrusions and an encircled heart logo stamped on its side. This sample was made mostly of plastic, because there wasn't any money or time to use titanium, the metal that would one day be used for fabrication. This was just a trial; the plastic would break down under stress, everyone knew, and the calf would die. The question was how long it would live before that happened.

Daniel's only job was to keep an eye on the Bivacor's console, which monitored blood flow, oxygen levels, and so on while sending operating instructions to the mechanical heart.

When Parnis was done, someone picked up the receiver from a wall phone and put in a call upstairs to Drs. Frazier and Cohn, who arrived looking a lot more relaxed than their Australian colleague. A tech crowned Billy with a light over his cap. Bud's burnt-orange University of Texas T-shirt showed yet again under his scrubs. Billy wore cowboy boots, while Bud had switched to some sort of clogs because of his aching knees. He had been putting off surgery for at least a year by that time, trying to ignore the pain but not really succeeding.

The implantation itself was relatively straightforward, given the magnitude of what it was supposed to do. Once the heart had been removed, the surgeons attached two fabric cuffs to the atria, the upper chambers of the heart that would be allowed to stay in place. They sewed two more cuffs onto the pathways to the lungs that would serve as connectors to tubes leading into the Bivacor. They connected the tubes to the device, and so on. It occurred to Daniel that this current iteration didn't seem much more advanced than something made in a backyard shed. He'd done all the wire prep and all the honing of the rotors himself.

This went on for a couple of hours, until Billy looked up from his work. His eyes met Bud's, both expressions expectant behind the men's masks. The heart was in. It was time to click the key on Daniel's keyboard and see if his invention was anything more than another well-designed but ultimately unworkable pipe dream. Daniel's fingertips were damp, and his breath shallow and humid beneath his mask.

Click one: levitation. Good, he thought, the impeller was suspended in its housing, floating on the flowing blood. Click two: rotation. Great, the Bivacor was beginning to spin, pushing the blood in one direction toward the lungs, and in the other outward into the rest of the body. The numbers in front of Daniel on the console looked good. The blood flow was five liters, a good amount for a calf. She was breathing fine. And the only sound coming from her chest—from the place where her heart should be—was a whispery, whirring whoosh of the blood being directed to the right places by a furiously spinning disc.

The fastest and most palpable pulse, in fact, was the one rushing through Daniel's temples. About three hours had passed. If the gods were on their side, the animal would wake up from the operation, and maybe even stand. That's all they needed to keep going.

The rest of the surgery—closing the chest, as in a human transplant—took another hour or so, and then the calf took a gurney ride to the animal ICU for recovery. The packed operating room emptied in an instant.

In the hallway outside, Bud snapped off his gloves and mask and threw them in the trash. Then he put on the white coat he had taken off to operate. He was pleased—he thought things had gone pretty well. He was already thinking ahead. "If this animal stands up," he said to no one in particular, "I'm going to take the result and I'm going to present it at the next International Society for Rotary Blood Pumps conference."

Of course it was too soon to tell, but Bud and Daniel strolled into the ICU for one last look at the calf before going their separate ways. About thirty minutes had passed since they had finished. She lay in a bed of hay in a small pen, resting quietly. Nearby, a couple of pigs snorted; a goat stood quietly in a stanchion. One of the vets and a small group of techs bustled about, checking on other animals, looking at monitors, recording results on clipboards.

Bud and Daniel had been standing there for about five minutes when the calf opened her eyes sleepily and then began to roll back and forth, slowly at first, and then *boom*! She was standing on all four legs. She blinked at the world around her with mild interest, including the two men staring back, openmouthed, unbelieving.

A few seconds passed before Daniel had the presence of mind to race over and grab his laptop, tapping into Skype as fast as he could to connect with his team, to show them the first living animal with a Bivacor instead of a heart. From Germany and Japan and Australia they stared goggle-eyed at their screens, clapping for what, if you didn't know what was going on, looked like a normal calf gazing back at them.

"Well," Bud said, allowing himself a small, wry grin, "I guess I'm going to conclude my talk with the device."

They named the calf Matilda, and she survived for a total of six hours with an artificial heart made of plastic, whirring and spinning in her chest.

—⋀⋀—

It was on that day that Billy knew what he had to do. The Bivacor had worked as he'd known it would. But Billy was a closet fretter, and its very success instilled a new fear: there was nothing tying Daniel to Houston except some newly won loyalty, and in the high-stakes world of medical devices that was no guarantee. Any company with a lot of cash could get wind of the Bivacor, and Daniel and his team could decamp. Then someone else would get all the credit for a discovery Billy was already comparing to a moon shot. But instead of from Houston, it would be launched from Cleveland or France or Tucson or somewhere else. Billy had to find more money, and fast.

The problem, as he and the whole THI team knew, was that funds for new medical devices were not easy to come by. In DeBakey's day, all you had to do was put on some fancy dog and pony show—after you'd cultivated friends in high places, of course—and millions in US government research funds could be yours. But those days were gone. And the bet-on-a-sure-thing mentality that governed public research had seeped into private giving as well. The venture capital types only wanted to invest in something they knew would pay off big-time—the second generation of an already successful drug was the kind of investment opportunity that really appealed. Private philanthropy too was drying up; the typical Houston givers wanted their names on opera halls and hospital donor walls. No one named a medical device after its investors.

Even in Houston, risk had become, if not a dirty word, then one that was more comfortably buttressed with lots of backup promises and mitigating assurances. Investors wanted proof, tests, predictable and successful outcomes. Whatever happened to those crazy Texas wildcatters, the ones willing to punch zillions of dry holes in the ground until they came up with a gusher? They had gone the way of leaded gasoline.

But then a name started muscling its way into Billy's consciousness: Jim McIngvale. Billy couldn't call him a close friend, exactly, but he did at least know him. Of course, just about everyone in town knew him, but by a slightly different name.

All cities have local celebrities, the kind of wealthy and colorful types whose fame never quite extends beyond local borders but thrives within them. Such a person was McIngvale, who was better known by his professional nickname, Mattress Mack. Think Crazy Eddie by way of Mississippi to Houston—with a bankruptcy thrown in for good measure—and you might have some idea of the person Billy had targeted: Mattress Mack had made a fortune selling what was essentially boomtown furniture—aspirational furniture, furniture for all the blue-collar workers who made Houston what it was when it was still a town of oil field workers and long-haul truckers, and then, later, furniture for all the immigrants from Zacatecas and Saigon and Mumbai and Karachi and Eritrea when oil started climbing again in the 1990s. Mack, as he was known to just about everyone, was a short, slight man with jug ears and an indeterminate southern accent whose frenetic energy in public belied a shrewd mind and a shy reserve—or simple exhaustion—in repose. He was

one of those 24/7 obsessives—"entrepreneurs" in local parlance—
that often seemed to make up at least 80 percent of Houston's population. Mack believed that customers who made around $50,000 a
year should be treated as well as hedge fund kings, which meant
that once you walked into a Gallery Furniture store, you didn't have
much chance of getting out without buying something. And so what
if you couldn't afford it? Instant financing was always available with
same-day delivery of your $2,500 American Heritage bedroom suite!

Founded in 1981, Mack's I-45 store was on its way to being the
single largest furniture emporium in the United States, and Mc-
Ingvale was much beloved because of his early, turbocharged TV
ads, in which he clutched wads of cash, jumped up and down, and,
in a Mississippi-on-meth kind of accent, promised that he would
"save . . . you . . . muh-neeee!" Sometimes McIngvale squeezed himself into a baby crib for the occasion. Supposedly he'd used his last
$10,000 to make his first crazy TV commercial in the oil boom
years of the early 1980s, another reason Mack was locally beloved
in a town where there was no shame in losing it all—as long as you
made it back. And, of course, Mack was generous in uniquely local
ways: he treated the homeless to a (branded) massive Thanksgiving
dinner, and he bought the grand champion steer at the charity auc-
tion sponsored by the Livestock Show and Rodeo. When the Rock-
ets won their first NBA championship in 1994, Mack paid for the
welcome-home party and waved to his grateful public from a float
in the victory parade. He stationed what he called the world's largest
Christmas tree outside one of his stores during the holidays.

Billy had met Mack in what was, for both of them, typical fashion. He was twenty-nine, finishing his fourth year of residency at
Baylor and working as a surgical chief resident at Ben Taub Hospital,
the huge charity hospital and trauma center that had just reopened
in a spanking-new building in 1990. Ben Taub was legendary in

Houston—the city had never been known for its generosity to the poor, and its public hospital had for decades been a pretty good example of a twentieth-century Bedlam. Thanks to a lack of public health clinics, most of Houston's poor used Ben Taub as their doctor's office, sometimes waiting days to be seen for common ailments. The hospital was also the only twenty-four-hour psychiatric facility in the city. But most important, Ben Taub was a level one trauma center. There was only one other in this city of 2.5 million, which meant that if you were stabbed or shot or in a horrific car accident, the ambulance was likely to take you there, where your chances of survival were the best in town. The place was staffed with Baylor-trained interns—DeBakey's shock troops—including, of course, Billy Cohn, who found himself perfectly at home. Operating on six to eight stab wounds a night, often without sleep, was his idea of nirvana.

But there was one big problem inside the gleaming new hospital: a shortage of furniture. Houston's glorious new monument to public healthcare had no place to put sick and injured patients who were awaiting transfers or X-rays or whatever. There were not enough gurneys, and there were not enough chairs for the people who had brought patients in to wait comfortably, away from the fray. Some crime victims found spots on hard plastic chairs, where they tried not to bleed on the brand-new vinyl flooring, but those who could move wandered off in search of more comfortable perches, and the staff, including the surgeons, lost precious hours roaming the hospital trying to track them down.

It was during such a search that the sleep-deprived Dr. William Cohn happened to catch a commercial on television of a man jumping up and down like one of Ben Taub's AWOL psychiatric patients. He seemed to be trying to sell recliners, because, he said, he had too many of them.

Soon after, without a nap or changing clothes—Billy did take a minute to throw a respectable white coat over his bloodstained scrubs—he got into his Toyota Celica and, jittery from sleeplessness and a jumbo-sized iced coffee, drove out of the Medical Center and headed north, past the gleaming towers downtown, and onto the congested lanes of I-45. The scenery was pretty squalid, a Houston hash of billboards and pawnshops and massage parlors and strip centers. He pulled off the freeway and into a place that looked like a giant circus tent. This was Gallery Furniture.

In the takes-one-to-know-one department, the meeting between Mattress Mack and Billy Cohn was something like Prince encountering David Bowie, or maybe P. T. Barnum meeting up with Wild Bill Hickok. Both were most comfortable operating at Mach speed, and both understood perfectly the uses of theater. (Mack's wife, Linda, often said that the two men lived by the same motto, which she described as "Shoot, ready, aim.") Mack listened patiently to Billy's rambling, somewhat incoherent plea. The county had run out of money, or maybe it was the city. Sick people were roaming around the hospital because there was no place to sit down in the waiting room. Ditto people with dying relatives. And, by the way, the interns had no place to sleep. Could Mack maybe possibly help them out with some recliners?

Mack's answer was swift, maybe because he was, by nature, a soft touch, or maybe because he wanted to get this lunatic in bloody clothes away from all that pristine furniture. Sure, OK. Mack had his workers fill up a moving truck with the recliners—about twenty at a total retail value of around $10,000—and deliver them to Ben Taub within seventy-two hours, free of charge.

The story might have had a happier, or at least more economical, ending if a hospital administrator hadn't noted that the recliners didn't meet the proper government standards for fire retardancy in healthcare facilities and ordered them returned. Mack had to order the correct recliners from Mississippi, which he then sent to Ben Taub—proof, perhaps, that no good deed goes unpunished.

That was that, until 2008, when Mack's beloved older brother George got very sick with congestive heart failure. He needed a pump—an LVAD—to keep him alive, and the surgeons best qualified to implant it were Dr. Bud Frazier and, yes, a better-rested and slightly longer-of-jowl Dr. Billy Cohn. Mack had not seen him in almost twenty years.

The surgeons were able to give George another few months of life, and then he lapsed into a coma. For six weeks he lay in the cardiac intensive care unit of the Texas Heart Institute, where Bud visited him night and day, on Thanksgiving, and on Christmas. It seemed to Mack that whenever he went to visit his brother, Bud was there or had just left, his large, lumbering frame perched onto the edge of the bed, his silver mane illuminated by the lights of the monitors in the darkened room, pinpoints of blue, red, and green like stars in some lonely alternate universe.

When the time came to take George off life support, Billy played bad cop, showing Linda X-rays of George's damaged heart, indicating that the machines were the only things keeping him alive. There was no hope. Bud guided the family to the final decision. The toughest one to convince was George's son, then a soldier on leave from a tour in Iraq, who refused to believe his father would not get better and go home. Bud met the young man by his father's bedside. "You're in the army, right?" he asked. Then he took the young man's hand and ran it up and down his father's sternum, grinding his knuckle as he applied pressure, the way medics do on the battlefield to test for any sign of pain or consciousness. There was nothing.

"You know what that means, right?" Bud asked. The young man nodded, surrendering.

George McIngvale was buried a few days later, after Christmas 2008. "We fought hard," Bud told Mack. "There were just too many bears in the woods."

Mack had never felt so grateful to anyone in his life. "Let me know if you ever need anything," he told the surgeons. It was that promise Billy Cohn would remember almost four years later.

—∿∿—

This time Billy drove up I-45 in a cobalt-blue, middle-age-crazy Audi R8 and significantly cleaner scrubs. His hairline had receded, but his energy level had not. A model of the Bivacor sat in a video camera bag on the passenger seat of the car.

In the ensuing years, Gallery Furniture had also undergone some changes. A fire set by an angry ex-employee had required a rebuild, and now the place looked like a supersized hamster cage, a sprawling, gargantuan human warren with tunnels and turrets. Several birdcages near the entrance featured parrots and macaws, and toy sports cars—not as nice as Billy's—that doubled as kid carriers sat parked nearby. There were, as always, red, white, and blue basketballs for the kids, and free slices of cake slumping under a heat lamp. The walls that weren't covered with photos of Mack—Mack and Linda; Mack and various generations of Bushes; Mack and pro basketball and football stars; and Mack in cowboy garb at the rodeo—trumpeted inspirational quotes, like "The only thing you get for nothing is failure." Myriad glass showcases displayed everything from Texas memorabilia to the basketball shoes of NBA stars.

And, of course, there was furniture, a dizzying array of it: cowhide rugs, bedroom sets, recliners, mattresses, even the occasional antique dresser. Mirrors and lamps set off by many, many scented candles. Sofas and fold-out sofabeds. Plastic slides in primary colors and mini-trampolines and basketball hoops for the kids' rooms. You needed a sack of bread crumbs to shop at Gallery and make it back to your car before nightfall.

Except, of course, for Billy, who was oblivious to his surroundings as he announced himself to the crew of salesmen who stood at the ready at the front desk. The bag containing the Bivacor was nearly weightless in his hands.

This time Mack was better prepared to ward off Billy's appeal. Like Billy, he had become something of a pitch magnet, and because he hated to say no, Mack often brought his wife along to keep him from saying yes to something stupid. Linda McIngvale had been her husband's adviser and enforcer since they had met in the late 1970s. Her devotion to Mack was not exactly of the Nancy Reagan total adoration variety, but it was just as ferocious—their bond had been forged after Jim had lost everything but Linda in a bankruptcy that had followed a youthful venture into the health club business. Unlike her husband, Linda was naturally ebullient, with long blondish hair and soft brown eyes that belied a mind every bit as sharp and hungry as her husband's. She wasn't flashy like a lot of rich Houston women: she usually skipped the makeup and favored jeans and Gallery Furniture polo shirts with her Prada bag.

The trio settled into a leather booth in the sunny Gallery employee cafeteria and Billy took the Bivacor out of the camera bag, holding it up to give the McIngvales a clear view. He explained that it could change the world—"This is the moon shot"—and Mack and Linda could be a part of that. He held the stubby little cylinder in his hands as if it were made of platinum instead of plastic. He opened it up, showed them the one moving part inside, and passed it to them for examination like a prop in a Billy Cohn magic show, which to some extent it was. He threw around terms that made Linda's head hurt, like "magnetic levitation" and "pulseless technology" and "hemato-something or other." Mack's eyes were flat; as he put it, "the ether had worn off" and he had pretty much decided this was a no-go for him. He understood scholarships for needy kids and feeding the homeless. Patriotism he got. He understood a lot about sports, and knew quite a bit about racehorses, because he owned some. But bio-medicine? Not his thing. "If you can convince my wife . . . ," he told Billy, Mack's way of signaling that he was inching toward the exit.

As a performer, Billy was sensitive to that moment when an audience started checking its collective watch. But he wasn't going back to the hospital empty-handed. OK, so what if he set up a meeting at the Texas Heart Institute? Give them a tour of the operating room? Introduce them to the boy genius, Daniel Timms? Reluctantly, the McIngvales agreed—mainly, again, to get Billy the hell out of the store. "You want me to go so I can be the one who says no," Linda said to her husband later.

Two things happened in the next few days. Linda got on the Internet and started reading about artificial hearts. Like her husband, she had only a high school education, but by that time it was fairly easy to find stories on Robert Jarvik and Barney Clark, on SynCardia and Rich Wampler. She noted how many people died of heart disease every year, and noted further how few hearts were available for transplants. She started writing things down and making lists of questions.

During the same period, Billy put in a call to Daniel, who was in Japan—to be exact, he was winding electrical coils by hand to make the motor for the next Bivacor.

Billy was breathless. "You gotta come back to Houston right now," he said.

As Daniel listened, his expression became one of exasperation and amazement. He was experiencing once more the essentials of Houston entrepreneurship.

Billy was still babbling. "I just went and talked with Mattress Mack," he said, sounding as if he had literally just left the room, which he probably had. Daniel was still groggy from the fifteen-hour time difference. He had only been in Japan for a few hours and had yet to unpack. In Billyworld, this was a good thing, as Daniel could quickly grab his bag and hop on a plane back to Houston.

"What's his name?" Daniel asked, trying to understand through the fog of his jet lag. "Mattress Mack?"

"He really wants to fund us," Billy explained. He sounded like a child begging his mother for Froot Loops at the grocery store.

Now Daniel was in familiar territory. "I've heard this a lot of times, Billy," he said, returning to the wires in his hands.

Two days later, Daniel was back on a plane, scheduled to meet the McIngvales at the Texas Heart Institute on December 13, 2012.

—⁄\/\—

The THI conference room could not be described as inviting. It is sprawling and windowless, its walls are covered in manly brown leather baffles. The wood floors are tinted a basketball court yellow and have been buffed to a high, almost blinding gloss. The gargantuan conference table is triangular in shape, echoing the light fixture that seems to hover above. It looks like the set of a *Star Trek* sequel, though it was actually the hospital brass' version of an auto showroom.

The McIngvales arrived in their usual dress—jeans and Gallery Furniture polo shirts. Dr. James Willerson, the eager, chatty president of THI, was there along with Dr. Denton Cooley. The ninety-two-year-old Cooley's skin was blotched and his hair was white, but his voice still crackled with electricity when he spoke. Bud and Billy were in scrubs; Daniel wore his jet lag. Mack would later tell a reporter for the *Chronicle*, perhaps a little disingenuously, that "there wasn't no doubt about who was the dumbest person in the room. Hands down."

People would later disagree about what exactly was said and what was promised, but this much was clear: Mack asked whether a donation from him might save the lives of people who had died like his brother. Willerson, the Grand Poo-bah of THI fundraising, answered in soft, satiny tones that, yes, quite possibly it could. Cooley's pitch was evocative of the successfully seductive tone he'd used on pretty nurses so many years ago. His eyes locked onto Mack's when he talked about the artificial heart. "This is my life's dream and I'd like to see it happen," he said.

Then Bud spoke, explaining that the device would work. He just knew it. Whereupon Billy and Daniel gave a presentation of the Bivacor, complete with animated slides depicting blood as floating blue and red dots moving in and out of the heart and lungs. Linda had questions, which surprised the men in the room more than any of them cared to admit. How was this device different from the LVAD, or from the artificial heart Robert Jarvik had invented? What about the French artificial heart, the Carmat? Or the one made by the company in Tucson, SynCardia?

Daniel explained that these were all conventional pumps of one sort or another, and that they would break or wear out too soon because they were pulsatile devices, or they were too big for anyone but large men, or they only addressed problems on the left side of the heart. They couldn't adjust, like the Bivacor, to the body's need for more blood at certain times. Daniel, like the other salesmen in the room, took her interest to be a good sign. Mack was harder to read, though he had teared up when Willerson had told him the device might have saved his brother.

Gradually, the talk wound around to how a donation might work—some might go to THI and some to the Bivacor. Tax advantages came up.

As it happened, Linda had brought along their checkbook. Well, hell, they had a little extra money at the time, and this sounded like a pretty good deal. She reached into her purse, took out her checkbook, and wrote out a check for $2.1 million. It was all the cushion they had, unless they wanted to sell a racehorse or their tennis club.

Later, while the McIngvales were waiting for the hospital valet to deliver their car, Billy tried to get Linda to watch him do a magic trick. He took five one-dollar bills and counted them out in his palm. Then, chattering away, he turned them over and counted them out again, and then caressed the bill on top with a slow stroke of his palm. When he showed Linda the money again, Ben Franklin was grimacing back at her from five $100 bills.

"I hate card tricks," Linda snapped. Card tricks were like drinking too much caffeine, she thought—if she saw one during the day, she'd stay up all night trying to figure out how it was done.

"I don't *do* anything," Billy told her, grinning so wide his molars sparkled. "It's magic."

THE OCCUPATION

Two million dollars may not have sounded like a lot of money to some people in 2012, but to Daniel Timms, it was as if his well had come in. After years of sleeping on couches, traveling with little more than a backpack, and communicating with his far-flung associates via Skype, he suddenly had a home for himself, his invention, and his team. His group was composed of fifteen or so mostly young, sunlight-deprived men from around the world, with heaviest representation from Japan, Germany, and Australia. There were hardware engineers to work on the machining of the Bivacor, software engineers who worked on the programming and interface of the device and the operating console, electrical engineers who worked on electrical components for the same, and experts in magnetic levitation charged with making sure the impeller inside the device spun at the proper velocity and in the proper spot. There was even, on occasion, a female veterinarian Daniel had worked with in Brisbane. Essentially, it was a team with everyone but the human medical experts, who came courtesy of THI. The Heart Institute had also arranged for the team's visas and paid for their transportation to Houston. It was the first time they had all been able to meet and work face-to-face in a single place.

Most of them settled in the dorm-like apartments near the Medical Center—the kind that featured fancy gyms, washers and dryers in each unit, party rooms, free Wi-Fi, and landscaped pools, everything that a single guy without a mom or girlfriend needed to function effectively. Thanks to Jim McIngvale—not for nothing was he called Mattress Mack—their apartments came completely furnished, free of charge.

The same was true of their workspace at the Texas Heart Institute, though that task was a lot more complex. Daniel's team got two rooms adjacent to the subterranean animal lab, one a clean, sterile space and one a conventional "dirty" space for more routine work. Up to that point, the Bivacor, such as it was, had been made elsewhere, and (compared to future models) fabricated of plastic, designed for a short life span for both the device and the animal who would host it. The prototype needed to last just long enough for testing purposes and, maybe, to impress a few investors.

There was a long way to go before Daniel and his team could produce something that would pass muster with the FDA. Not only would they have to create a finished machine—its design "frozen," in industry parlance—they would also have to prove that it could be manufactured and marketed on a mass scale without any hiccups, or worse. That is, they would have to avoid the kind of production and usage problems that had plagued the Hemopump. The process would not be cheap: the average cost of bringing a device like the Bivacor to market had also been steadily rising, largely due to the ever-increasing caution of the FDA and the relentlessness of plaintiffs' lawyers. All told, Daniel would eventually need to come up with about $75 million just to get the agency's approval. McIngvale's contribution, then, was the first big drop in a very deep bucket.

Still, the team was off to a good start. The basement space, built in the seventies and looking pretty much like a high school chemistry classroom, with fluorescent lighting and battered wood cabinets, was swiftly upgraded to the twenty-first century. Along with all sorts of computers and electronic devices with multiple gauges that looked mysterious, the battered, black-topped tables now hosted mock circulation loops, a series of tall, narrow plastic cylinders and piping connected to computer terminals. When everything was switched on, they pulsed and bubbled with fluid, resembling fancy tablescapes for an oil field equipment gala. In fact, they were miniaturized replicas of the human circulatory system. Many calves would be spared, and money saved, thanks to the machines: the loops were a first line of defense, enabling the engineers to see how adjusting the pump's speeds and pressures would work inside the body. There were loops for the left side of the heart and for the right.

Computers with specialized software for drawing models and producing the specific calculations to build them had also been on Daniel's shopping list, and now here they were. They would be used to refine the design for, among other things, the impeller, that part of the centrifugal pump that directed the way the blood spun on its path. (Imagine the center of an old-fashioned washing machine, but instead of swishing and agitating dirty clothes, the impeller spins blood to the proper destination.) What worked best to prevent clotting, for instance? Should the impellers be taller or shorter, wider or narrower? A combination of both? How tall should each be and how far apart should they be spaced to make sure the blood couldn't clot in between? Did one shape work better for the left side of the heart and another for the right? Now the engineers could design and redesign to their heart's content without making a dent in the bovine population of Texas.

More calves would be saved, thanks to the machine in the adjacent "dirty" room, the crown jewel of the new lab: a 3-D printer. An invention of the 1980s, it stacked layers of a fluid that turned solid when it came in contact with ultraviolet light, duplicating whatever it "saw" into a replica in three dimensions.

The machine was a success from the moment it hit the market: the more expensive ones could copy highly technical car and airplane parts for industry, or medical devices like artificial heart valves and artificial knees to replace worn-out human ones. A 3-D printer for home use could make anything from soap dishes to coffee cup sleeves to doorstops to kids' action figures to handguns. Prices for these printers ranged anywhere from $125 to $2,500 on amazon.com.

The Bivacor team's copier was about the size of a dishwasher and cost in the tens of thousands of dollars. Almost as soon as it arrived, someone printed out a mini version of the Eiffel Tower with all the lacy metalwork reproduced in a shimmering, inky black. Within days, it was fabricating plastic Bivacor models in near-infinite variations.

Almost as crucial for symbolic reasons was a tall, narrow glass case just inside the clean lab. It's the kind you see in jewelry or eyeglass stores, with transparent sides and shelves. The contents would have been completely unidentifiable to a layperson but, for the informed, served as a constant reminder of how rocky and arduous the path of progress can be. In it, an old Liotta pump sat next to a Jarvik-7. The 1985 issue of *Life* magazine with a cover photo of William DeVries and William Schroeder sat on the shelf above. There was a tiny Hemopump, octopus-like with the tubes still attached, and two LVADs pieced together, similar to what went in Craig Lewis' chest. Once so radical, these devices were gathering dust now.

But for Bud, the artifacts, the lab, and all the new lab equipment served as a continuation of the path he'd been on since he'd been a med student, squeezing the heart of a helpless boy to keep him alive. He could never quite believe that so many of the things he or a colleague had done by hand could now be done by machine—Robert Jarvik and Richard Wampler had done all their schematic drawings with pen and paper, after all, as no computer software existed at the time to help them hone the size, shape, or efficacy of their devices. Fabrication that had once taken months could now be done nearly overnight—all refinements programmed in, all mistakes repaired.

As usual, Bud converted the near incomprehensibility of such awesome technological progress into a story. He told it to anyone who would listen, but mostly he was telling it to himself. Just back from Vietnam in 1969, the story went, he had headed to West Texas to see his ninety-four-year-old grandfather. When the two got to talking about recent events, Bud's grandfather mentioned that the moon landing a few months back had never happened. "They faked it," he insisted. The two men bantered until they were bickering, and then the argument grew heated, as Bud declared he could not believe his grandfather was being so willfully ignorant. Finally the old man gave up: after all, he'd lived long enough to see airplanes soar over the same vast, empty land he'd once crossed on horseback while driving cattle across the Panhandle. "Well, maybe it happened," Bud's grandfather finally admitted of the moon landing. "But I'd rather not think about it."

Sometimes that was how Bud felt too. The Bivacor amazed and thrilled him, but when it came to the minutiae of data points and CAD software, he'd rather leave that work to younger men. Age and experience had taught him that the machines changed, but the heart stayed the same, its most important secrets still tantalizingly close and yet infinitely far away.

—∿—

One way to tell when Bud was in one of his darker moods was to check the movies running on his office television. You didn't want to make too much of things, as sometimes he just left the thing set to Turner Classic Movies for hours, but too many Russian films with English subtitles could be an indicator. Also, he wasn't by nature a complainer—male heart surgeons, along with aged West Texas grandfathers, were experts at not only denial but compartmentalization— and normally he didn't have much to complain about, since there were so many people in his life charged with making sure he could save as many lives as possible without distractions. So it was noticeable when he started making cracks about THI management and asking why the once jammed parking lot at St. Luke's suddenly had an abundance of spaces. It didn't seem possible that anything could throw him off his game, but it was clear something had.

The trouble had started right around the time Daniel had arrived, toward the end of 2012. Bud's faith in the Bivacor was unshakable, and the new opportunity to develop it should have, if anything, made him feel a part of something boldly new, a rarity for someone in his eighth decade. But Bud had also lived for more than forty years in a world of his own making, reinforced at every turn by the elite culture of the Texas Heart Institute and, for that matter, the Texas Medical Center. An expert in those manners and folkways, Bud was especially sensitive to any changes in the local atmosphere. He knew too that the world of medicine was perpetually changing—he groused about it, like all doctors—but he couldn't have perceived how swiftly and relentlessly change could come to his own protected corner of the world.

But come it did. The ever-growing cost of medical care was causing titanic shifts in the profession and its attendant businesses; sensible people knew that preventive care was the best path forward in all healthcare, including that for heart disease. But preventive care wasn't profitable. Research and innovation were nice too, but they were expensive and the payoff slow and unpredictable; the big money was in really sick people who had to be hospitalized. In turn, the best hospitals, of course, wanted the best doctors to attract patients. All of these theoretical issues soon became grim realities for Bud and the stellar career he had built for himself in Houston.

The first sign of trouble occurred when a new CEO of one particular Houston hospital chain began aggressively picking off some of the best heart surgeons at THI: with Cooley aging out, there were plenty of midcareer surgeons who were open to offers of more money and spiffier new facilities down the road. Other longtime colleagues and staffers chose retirement over adapting to a change that was surely coming. The next chief of cardiovascular surgery could not probably command his own photographer, for instance. Bud wasn't the kind of guy to stand in anyone's way, but suddenly there were fewer people to work with and jaw with around St. Luke's. That he had recruited and mentored so many of them meant that Bud couldn't help but take the departures personally. They didn't want the life he had led—the hospital as home, the drama and exhaustion of twenty-four-hour days, saving the lives of others as the ultimate proof of their own value.

But that was just the beginning. Baylor Medical School, where Bud had been on the faculty for more than three decades, came under new management after a spate of inept leadership in DeBakey's wake. (One recent former president married his second wife in Las Vegas after his abrupt departure. The two wore matching gold lamé jumpsuits for the ceremony, resulting in a viral photograph that delighted the Baylor docs who had been suspicious of his competence and intent during his tenure.) The decline of Baylor, of course, meant a decline in Bud's own currency, like any other doctor on the faculty. He was incensed when the new president accepted a $100 million-dollar gift from the owner of the local NFL franchise to build yet another hospital. Bud hoped the money would go to medical research, but research didn't pay.

Now Baylor too had a hospital to fill with stars, and its leadership began working overtime to lure, and then muscle, the Baylor doctors who had been working around town to move into the new facility. The Texas Heart Institute surgeons were high on their shopping list. With another potential exodus on the horizon, Bud began referring to the new place as "that empty hospital" or "that hospital with no doctors."

But the biggest shock came in May 2013. Rumors had been circulating for months that the Episcopal Diocese of Texas, which had founded St. Luke's in 1954, had decided to get out of the hospital business, particularly with the anticipated changes coming under President Barack Obama's Affordable Care Act. Like a lot of people in and around the Medical Center, Bud was hoping for a merger with DeBakey's beloved affiliate, Methodist Hospital. St. Luke's and Methodist were both the medical equivalent of five-star hotels, after all; the combination of their cardiothoracic teams would mean Houston had more than a fighting chance to recover some of the former glory it had been losing over the years to the Cleveland Clinic, which was now the leader in heart health in the United States.

Instead, the diocese shocked both the medical community and the community at large by selling St. Luke's to the highest bidder, a Colorado conglomerate called Catholic Health Initiatives, or CHI, which had $2 billion in hand and was eager to move into the Texas market. Initially, it wasn't clear whether THI was part of the deal or not; since its inception in 1962, the Institute had never been owned or governed by St. Luke's. A simple affiliation—the Texas equivalent of a handshake deal, in essence—had worked to the mutual benefit of both for decades. St. Luke's got the considerable income generated from the surgical stars at Texas Heart Institute, while the doctors at THI got access to the high-dollar patients streaming in the door. Everyone was happy.

Now, however, THI found itself in the situation of a spoiled mistress whose sugar daddy had suddenly skipped town, to be replaced with a stern Catholic priest. Bud was as shocked as anyone to learn that no one had been looking too closely at the books for St. Luke's or THI: both had been operating under massive debt—$20 million in the case of THI, whose president at the time, James Willerson, had been doling out massive amounts of cash to attract and keep medical heavy hitters from all over the United States. Willerson, who had been an enthusiastic presence during the Bivacor presentation to the McIngvales, had become particularly infatuated with the latest, edgiest trend in cardiac advances, stem cell research: finding a way to teach a damaged heart to regenerate healthy cells and repair itself.

It didn't bode well that both Denton Cooley and Bud Frazier learned of the St. Luke's sale the way most ordinary Houstonians did—by reading about it in the newspaper.

—∿—

For Bud, all this change meant that by early 2014, walking from the parking garage into St. Luke's and the Texas Heart Institute was like entering territory controlled by an occupying army. CHI was eager to put its stamp on its new purchase, and set about doing so by unveiling the obligatory multimillion-dollar rebranding campaign for the new entity, CHI St. Luke's Health. Now there were cheery billboards, full-page newspaper ads, and banners in the hospital's public spaces declaring "the dawn of a new era in health" and urging new and old patients to "imagine" all sorts of things related to wellness, as opposed to scary things like heart disease.

Another campaign followed several months later, called "Living Proof," which was supposed to tout CHI's new, deeper affiliation with Baylor. This campaign featured the cardiologists and heart surgeons from the Texas Heart Institute (many of whom were also

Baylor professors) showing off their innovations, along with the patients who were "living proof" of their success. Bud was prominently featured in print ads and TV commercials, talking about transplants and LVADs with all his medical titles prominently highlighted—Professor of Surgery at Baylor, Chief of Transplant Services at Baylor St. Luke's Medical Center, and Director of Surgical Research, Texas Heart Institute. He held a Bivacor in his hand, though most people probably had no idea what it was. "Why trust your heart to anyone else?" the ad asked.

But CHI's commitment only went so far. Historically, the chain had been devoted to community healthcare, with little interest—despite their ad campaign—in surgical innovation or research. Nor was it a chain of big spenders: the once pristine stairways of St. Luke's grew grimy and spotted with trash. Bud tried to interest the new leadership in the storied history of THI by giving them copies of a 1973 Cooley biography, but these people were not interested in any legacy but their own.

Then there was the fundraiser in honor of Bud's thirty years of service in the spring of 2014. There had been a big blowout on THI's fiftieth anniversary in 2012, a black-tie fundraiser in Cooley's honor. Lyle Lovett played a set, and James Baker III delighted the crowd with jokes about Cooley's tightness with a dollar. Texas governor Rick Perry showed up, and there were video tributes from former presidents Bill Clinton and George H. W. Bush. Bud's, in contrast, had a thrown-together quality. He had never expected a big bash like Cooley's, but he had hoped his three decades would be recognized in a way that acknowledged the importance of his accomplishments at THI. The venue was elegant enough—another luxury hotel ballroom. And Cooley was present, along with a few hundred friends and colleagues. But many of the people Bud was closest to couldn't get tickets because the room was small or because the notice had been short. There was a fight over who would get the majority of the money raised that night, CHI or THI. There was little reflection of the rich and varied life Bud had brought to bear on his practice. There was no music from Lyle Lovett—who probably would have shown, given that Bud had kept the folk music venue that gave him his start from going under. There were no words of praise from writers he admired and had become close to, like Mary Karr or Larry McMurtry, whom Bud had advised on his heart problems. Not even a video from Dick Cheney, though Bud had consulted on the implantation of his LVAD. There were no appearances, either, from people Bud had helped in far-flung places like Afghanistan and the Middle East. In his introduction, the head of CHI talked mostly about the company's goals. His speech had all the intimacy of a eulogy delivered at a funeral by a minister who didn't know the deceased.

Billy Cohn wasn't thrilled with the changes at Texas Heart Institute either, but he kept himself occupied, or, as was so often true in Billy's case, overly occupied. Throughout his medical career, he had always been as interested in making things that made surgery easier and safer as he had in actually operating on people. By 2014, in fact, he had close to eighty patents awarded or pending. He continued to win major prizes too, including a highly coveted silver Edison Award in 2013 for the SentreHEART LARIAT, a tiny, magnetized loop that could be threaded through the body via cardiac catheterization to tie off a small, useless protrusion of heart muscle thought to be a danger to those with an irregular heartbeat. (Billy, of course, fretted that he hadn't won the gold.) Like many other inventions created by

Cohn, this one reduced the need for open-heart surgery. Billy was also spending a lot of time in Paraguay, where he was working with a team to create an easier, nonsurgical entry port for dialysis patients.

When he wasn't inventing—or even while he was inventing—Billy served on the board of several medical device companies, and was busy creating others. The failure of his early reality show was long forgotten; Billy had evolved into an innovation evangelist, a brilliant spokesperson and salesperson not only for his own devices but for the Texas Heart Institute. He knew how to reduce the arduousness of invention to a lively after-dinner speech; in fact, he could make building a total artificial heart sound like a simple matter of buying the right stuff at Home Depot and putting the pieces together over a weekend. It didn't matter whether he was performing in front of a high school or college science class, a tiny if adoring women's club, or a major inventors' organization; Billy strutted and pivoted and paced across the stage, as excited and flamboyant as a medical Mick Jagger.

"We can't afford to take care of our sick," Billy preached. "The key to fixing all our healthcare problems is . . . innovation." He'd move on to cite the great inventors—Thomas Edison, Nikola Tesla, et cetera—and tell the hoary story about DeBakey and his trip to the department store to make the Dacron graft that changed heart history. (It was always new to someone.) You had to notice unmet needs. You had to ignore the naysayers ("Just because everybody tells you it won't work . . . do it anyway"). You had to recognize your frustrations: "There's always an opportunity to mitigate frustration," he'd say. Why, he invented a foot pedal for his refrigerator door because he hated trying to open it when his hands were full.

What Billy didn't say is that it also helped to be Billy, whose determination matched his stratospheric IQ and boundless curiosity, as well as his unceasing, perpetually powered drive.

These qualities did not go unnoticed beyond THI. Most medical innovation these days comes from enormous multinational corporations like Medtronic and Johnson & Johnson, who have the billions required to bring multiple products to market—and to buy smaller companies that develop them. It so happened that in 2014 Billy was on a plane to Tel Aviv for yet another medical conference, and he found himself seated next to an old friend, Bruce Rosengard. Rosengard, a tall, supremely confident heart surgeon and inventor, was Johnson & Johnson's chief science and medical technology officer. On that particular day, he had a pressing problem. The corporation wanted to put an innovation center in the Texas Medical Center and build relationships with the local hospitals. The TMC was visited by about ten million patients a year, many of whom might be interested in participating in clinical trials for new medicines and new devices. But Rosengard hadn't been able to find the right person to head the venture. He needed someone dynamic. Someone who was a great medical innovator, but who also knew all the players in Houston.

By the end of the flight, he was pretty sure he had his man.

THE POWER SOURCE

By the beginning of 2016, a sense of urgency to try the Bivacor started overtaking just about everyone but Daniel Timms. "I'd put it in a patient today if I could," Bud would say. He was that sure. He would have done an emergency implantation, like the kind they had done on Lewis, as winning FDA approval for an emergency, lifesaving experiment took almost no time at all. They could work out the bugs afterward.

Bud had been around this particular engineer-versus-physician mulberry bush before: guys like Daniel wanted to make a pump that would allow a patient to play a mean game of tennis, while Bud knew that lots of folks just wanted to be able to walk across a room. Of course, the FDA only gave you two shots at experimental use—that's one reason he was no longer working on the twin Heart-Mate device. That and the fact that Bud was so sure Daniel's Bivacor would work infinitely better.

Bud ached to try it. People were sick and in need, and coincidentally or not, success with the Bivacor would also ensure the importance of continuous flow, Bud's legacy. If he wished he had come up with the idea himself, he didn't show it. Bud bragged about the Bivacor to colleagues and friends like a father whose child had been accepted to every Ivy League school. He knew it would work, he just knew it.

Billy too was ready to move on to the next step—or jump ahead several. He was interested in the Johnson & Johnson gig but he wasn't sure about giving up surgery, and he had no intention of giving up on the Bivacor. Still, experience told him that $2 million wouldn't go very far, and he had begun chatting up investors in Houston, Austin, and beyond, using the term "one moving part"—one of the Bivacor's defining features—like a mantra.

There was certainly reason to be optimistic. Thanks to the money, they had been able to switch from fragile plastic to durable titanium devices as often as they needed to. Calf study after calf study went well—within a couple of years they had done almost a dozen—with calves easily living the FDA requisite of ninety days. (At that point, they "sacrificed the animal," in the delicate parlance of the lab.) During that time, the calves demonstrated that they could not only wake up and stand and rummage in a brightly colored bucket for snacks, but move easily on a veterinary treadmill with "Good Horsekeeping" emblazoned on its side. The initial goal was five minutes on the treadmill, which then lengthened to eight minutes, ten minutes, and more. The starts could be rocky—in the beginning the calf might lean to one side and then the other, tuckered out. But soon enough he or she began to stroll easily, if not for too long, while the accompanying group of humans jubilantly called out respiratory rates and cardiac output—the number of liters of blood pumped from the heart. Almost from the beginning, those numbers were within normal range, from five to seven liters a minute.

The software-driven miracle that separated the Bivacor from many other devices was also proven time and again: if the animal sped up, the machine pumped more blood throughout its body. If the calf slowed down, the Bivacor took a breather, just like the heart did in normal humans.

But there was always another unknown. "What happens if the animal is frightened?" someone asked Bud one day. "Will the heart speed up then too?" After all, that happened to a human heart if someone was, say, held up in an alley or caught sight of a person he had a desperate crush on.

Bud looked flummoxed, and for just a moment took his eyes off the animal strolling steadily on the treadmill, extending its soft black muzzle in search of a treat Billy was holding just out of reach. "I don't know," he said. "Let's ask Daniel."

He stepped over a few wires and tubes to saunter over to the spot where Daniel had his eyes fixed on the computer console. Well, what about it? he asked Daniel. Would the Bivacor pump more blood if the calf was scared?

For just a second Daniel looked up from his screen with what was for him the rarest of expressions: surprise. "I never thought about that," he said.

Precisely for that kind of reason—all the myriad things he might not have thought of, or, more likely, all the things he knew he could make better—Daniel resisted the Cohn/Frazier push for a human implantation. He continued to work painstakingly and methodically to make sure his machine was as close to flawless as he could make it. Maybe if the prongs on the impeller were just a little farther apart or a little closer together, the blood flow could be even better. Maybe they needed more or fewer data points than twenty thousand to keep the center of the device magnetically spinning without touching the sides and causing wear that could lead to bigger problems.

Not that he couldn't see the future himself. Daniel began traveling to San Diego, where he had found a manufacturer—one who mass-produced pumps for Thoratec and other companies that were now cleaning up on LVADs. Daniel's Facebook page filled up with pretty Pacific sunsets.

—∿—

There was another reason Daniel was spending more time out of town. He was beginning to experience a different curriculum in his education in innovation, or, to put it another way, his initial sense of awe at all he had been given was gradually being eroded by inventors' paranoia. He was starting to worry about losing control of his creation. Several alarming superhighways could lead to this dangerous destination. Someone could copy it, or borrow enough of the technology to get to market faster, or, as had happened with Wampler and the Hemopump, he could find himself at the mercy of his investors. They could lose interest, something that was not uncommon with venture capitalists, or they could clutch the purse strings even tighter while demanding a larger ownership share. They could object if the pool of investors got too big and diluted both their power and their possible return. Helping humankind was certainly part of the process, but very few people invest large sums without also expecting a big payday down the road.

Keeping the particulars of the device secret wasn't such a big problem. Daniel started banning cellphones from the implantations—no more selfies with the bionic calves—and he also started limiting the number of people allowed to witness the surgeries, period. If someone asked to listen to the Bivacor's whooshing inside a calf's chest and that someone wasn't a medical professional or an investor, Daniel just said no.

But keeping up a charm offensive with investors was not as easy,

particularly because Daniel didn't have much patience with or interest in people who did not come from his world. Indeed, by January 2016 a couple of fissures were appearing in his relationship with
the McIngvales. The problem dated back to what had been said at
that first meeting at THI in 2012, specifically whether the fabled
$2 million from the couple was an investment in the Bivacor, a
charitable donation to be channeled through the Heart Institute, or
maybe a little of both. Fundraising, like operating, had always been
done somewhat on the fly at Texas Heart; Cooley or Bud or someone
else put in a phone call to someone with a lot of money or power and
somehow it all worked out.

But now, as the disparate interest groups—some of them new
to the story—tried to formalize their agreement, it became unclear
whether, for instance, Billy in his eagerness had promised the Mc-
Ingvales something he didn't have the authority to deliver. It was unclear what, exactly, THI's role was in all of this—were they going to
be the recipient of a philanthropic windfall, or was it all supposed to
go to the Bivacor? The fact that the Heart Institute had been without
a CEO since the CHI takeover contributed to the problems; no one
could make a decision.

As time went on, the McIngvales also became concerned about
sharing the Bivacor with new investors. Billy had found a Texas
venture capital firm that was eager to throw $5 million in the pot,
but the couple was not enthused about diluting their interest, and
neither was Bud, whose suspicion of venture capitalists dated back
to the homicide of the Hemopump. He would have preferred more
government grants, assuming any existed. As for Daniel, he had terrified everyone involved by suggesting he might take an open-ended
trip back to Brisbane.

The only certainty was this: suddenly everyone, including Daniel,
was lawyered up, and everyone was pointing fingers at everyone else.
It was Jim McIngvale who proposed a peace dinner at Del Frisco's

Double Eagle Steakhouse, a Houston favorite. Located in the high-end Galleria shopping mall, it had the feel of a dealmaker's paradise, with dry-aged steaks, dim if flattering lighting, leather banquettes, and, all-important in ultra-casual Houston, no requirement of a coat and tie.

Bud was out of town at a conference; Billy brought the affable Mishaun; Daniel brought his second in command, an electrical engineer by the name of Nick Greatrex, a pensive, bearded Australian who managed to be both warmer and quieter than Daniel. Jim brought Linda, though whether her role that night was as human shield or bad cop was not immediately clear. She wore a pair of unpretentious reading glasses atop her long blond hair, and, like her husband, jeans and a polo shirt embroidered with the Gallery Furniture name. The McIngvales also had a son-in-law in tow whose dress and manner suggested more than a passing acquaintance with a solid MBA program.

At first there was a lot of friendly chitchat of the sort designed to flatter the most important person at the table, even if he was the host. There was, for instance, a discussion of an Arab sheik who was on his way to Houston to look at one of Mack's racehorses for possible purchase. This was followed by much hilarity over some vibrating test beds Mack had given Billy and Daniel that hadn't worked so well. Billy did an imitation of a man folded up in a shaking rollaway. "I told him not to do it," Linda said, shaking her head at her husband in triumph.

Finally Billy reached down under his seat and pulled up a small black box with silver trim, a combination lock, and the word "Vaultz" stamped on it. He placed it atop the white tablecloth with the flair of the magician he was and opened it to reveal . . . the latest iteration of the Bivacor. This one was made of titanium with a brushed chrome-like finish, and sported four stubby legs protruding from a squat cylinder stamped with the Bivacor logo, a valentine-like heart inside a circle. It was at least 30 percent smaller than the earlier models, closer now to the size of a golf ball than, say, a baseball. If you didn't know what it was, you might think it was some sort of car part that went somewhere around the air filter. When Billy challenged the tuxedoed waiter to guess its purpose, the young man looked panicky, like a kid who got called on when he hadn't done his homework. "It's gonna change the world," Billy told him. Then he showed the Bivacor to the people sitting at the next table and told them the same thing.

Billy passed the Bivacor around the table and everyone held it gently, as if it were made of the finest crystal instead of hefty metal. He was, he said, beyond optimistic. Thanks to Mack and Linda, he added, they had been able to get twice as much done in two-thirds the time. Another calf implant was scheduled in two months, and soon they were going to take the first steps toward FDA approval by doing the required eight animal implants, each exactly the same. "How long will that take?" Linda asked, a crease forming between her brows.

"With the next $5 million we will start the GLP studies," Billy said, moving on to discuss the standardized quality control system— good laboratory practice—the government required.

"Why does that take $5 million?" Mr. MBA asked, which was certainly a reasonable question.

Well, Billy explained with none of the testiness he sometimes showed his underlings, they would soon have to go out to other companies to get help refining the design for mass production. They needed input from software engineers, hardware engineers, experts in electronics to make it the best it could be. There would no doubt be many more refinements.

Billy was rolling now. You almost expected him to say, "Pick a card, any card." It was a good time to bring up the bad news: they were running out of money when there was still so much more to do. "All I gotta do is get this across the goal line and then I'll sit on the beach and play Words with Friends," he declared—an unlikely scenario, particularly because he was in the process of talks with Johnson & Johnson, a topic that did not come up.

The large, sizzling steaks arrived, along with generous bowls of glistening creamed spinach, golden potatoes au gratin, colossal onion rings, and just about anything else that could be considered a required side dish in a steakhouse. The talk of calf experiments didn't seem to diminish anyone's appetite.

Across the table, Daniel looked thoughtful and sphinx-like. "What do y'all think of the name Bivacor-Timms Heart?" Billy asked, eyeing Daniel as he cut into his dinner.

"You get this thing to work, you can call it poop if you want," Linda responded.

"I like the Biva-*Cohn*," Billy cracked, keeping all the happy plates spinning. He chuckled, and everyone, including Daniel, smiled at him indulgently.

"You know," Mack said, "they oughta do a reality show on you." Then he turned serious. "Tell me," Mack said, fixing his eyes on Billy. "How many lives is the heart gonna save?"

There wasn't really a good answer to that question, but Billy punted, citing the number of possible recipients as "millions."

Mack turned to fix a level gaze on Daniel. "Daniel, how much more money do you need?" he asked.

No time elapsed before the answer. "Four hundred grand a month for eighteen months," he said, without a trace of anxiety. The Aussie was becoming more Texan by the minute.

Of course, Billy added hurriedly, they would need at least $15 million *more* for a human study. "And then," he said, chewing furiously, "the value goes through the roof."

In fact, he already had several other angels interested in investing.

"I've been involved in a lot of projects," he added. "I've never been involved in a project where *everybody* wants in."

Linda's face clouded up again. "What are the terms?"

"Exact terms as you," Billy said with a shrug, cutting into his steak again.

"What are you valuing the company at today?" she pressed.

"Twenty million flat," Billy said. A venture capital firm in Austin was desperate to invest. "They are *pounding* us," he said.

Linda asked to see a budget sheet and a business plan for the next phase. "Try to find investors we approve of," she said quietly.

Billy nodded, but something else was pinching at his enthusiasm. "It's imperative that we have it in a person while Bud is still standing," he declared, "it" being the Bivacor. Everyone nodded in agreement, and no one laughed.

There was no specific thing to point to, when it came to Bud's aging. He seemed reasonably healthy. Often, when someone asked how he was, he would joke, "I'm better, thank you," which made the person asking wonder what he had missed, which was usually nothing. Still, the stress of the regime change was beginning to take its toll, and on particularly bad days, Bud would give in to self-pity, claiming that his only remaining goal was to see the Bivacor through to human trials, a date he set for about two years hence.

And then, he got a call from Los Angeles on a spring day in March 2016. His beautiful daughter, Allison, forty-five, who was happily married with a young son and a daughter, had to have emergency surgery—doctors had discovered a tumor in her bowel. Rachel was already packing for California. Bud kept trying to pretend it was an ordinary day—working on an introduction for a new book about pumps (*Circulatory Assistance and the Artificial Heart*), telling a story about a medical conference in Moscow ("We'd present something, then the Russians would present something that looked like a high school science project"), but he couldn't quite pull it off. It was as if his ability to compartmentalize was finally failing him, maybe a function of age, or something else.

There were interruptions from his assistant, Libby, who kept giving him updates as she continued trying to get him on the earliest possible flight. There were calls from a former student Bud had contacted for referrals for Allison. She was now a prominent surgeon who was also an author with her own TV series on the heart, which seemed to make Bud contemplate his own path once more.

He made it to California and refused to stay at the hotel, choosing instead to park himself at the hospital before, during, and after his daughter's surgery. When Allison talked about her successful operation later, it was her father she talked most about—how present he was for her, checking her chart and her meds, asking the right questions, pushing for answers, making sure nothing went wrong. If he had missed so many years of her life saving others, he was certainly there for her now.

Despite Billy and Bud's hopes, the team had one big hurdle to clear, the one that would forever distinguish the Bivacor from its competitors: a sustainable power source that functioned inside the body. The pacemaker, which regulated abnormal heart rhythms, was such a fully implantable device, to use the lingo of the medical professionals. But no LVAD was, as yet, and neither was the SynCardia artificial heart, that updated version of the old Jarvik-7. They all still required an external power source, a battery pack that recipients can tuck into specially designed shoulder bags. This situation was not ideal for several reasons. First, any tubes or wires going in and out of the body are prime sites for infection—just ask anyone who is stuck wearing a catheter. Second, the battery packs looked like any purse or man bag, especially to thieves. Jarvik recalled one patient who fell victim to purse snatchers, collapsing as soon as the drive lines in their bags were snapped away by the miscreants. Third, the batteries didn't last long enough. A patient with a flat tire or any other minor inconvenience could suddenly find herself in a dire situation if she didn't have a spare battery or enough time to get home to recharge.

The main reason an implantable power source doesn't exist is that for decades there was no reason to develop one. A heart assist device that only lasted two years or so didn't need a battery that could last for ten. Where was the incentive in that? But as the LVADs improved in durability, and particularly as continuous flow replaced pulsatile pumps, the need suddenly appeared on the horizon. Once Daniel and his team got closer to freezing the design of the actual pump—FDA-speak for Daniel to stop tinkering—they would have to start thinking about new ways to power his invention. The optimum solution, of course, would be something self-contained inside the body.

This was not a new idea. In 1967, before the implantation of the artificial heart in Haskell Karp, and long before Barney Clark was driven nearly mad by the pounding of the enormous air compressor keeping his heart pumping—that is, when faith in the artificial heart was still unshakable—the US government and several big engineering companies were certain they could find a way to power the artificial heart internally. The energy generator of choice? Plutonium-238.

It probably made a lot of sense at the time. After all, back in the sixties, Michael DeBakey had set a ten-year deadline for the artificial heart. It was quickly decided by various government, corporate, and medical experts that the only way to power such a device—to compete with the natural heart's 120,000 beats a day for, say, twenty to thirty years or more—was to, literally, go nuclear. At the time, no ordinary battery lasted more than several hours. A short-term internal power source guaranteed a ticket back to the ER for open-heart surgery.

Enlightened self-interest also played a role. The US government, in the guise of the Atomic Energy Commission, was eager to put a positive spin on what had been a very ugly experiment—the nuclear research that evolved into the weapon that forced the Japanese surrender in World War II. Engineering firms like Westinghouse Electric and McDonnell Douglas were also eager to apply what they had learned in wartime toward commercial use—especially when Uncle Sam was offering to dole out a total of $14 million (or about $300 million in today's dollars) to pay for the research. Willem Kolff was one of many inventors lobbying for the effort. In fact, just about everyone involved was on board with the nuclear option, including researchers at the Texas Heart Institute.

The research lab created by Dr. John Norman in 1972—Cooley's big recruit from Harvard, who lived with his Great Dane in the lab—did a lot of work but came up with very little. Norman's pump was sponsored by the National Heart, Lung, and Blood Institute, which was competing with another sponsored by the Atomic Energy Commission in an intragovernmental contest. Powered by a thermal converter fueled by plutonium, it was supposed to make the heart run like a steam engine, converting fluid to vapor. The plutonium was secured inside three different capsules to prevent any leakage.

No adequate power source would emerge from this work, or anyone else's, partly because there wasn't really any effective artificial heart or assist device at the time. By 1977, the whole enterprise was dead because the government had withdrawn its support, partly due to financial concerns and partly because the public had become much more skeptical of the artificial heart itself. Even before the frightening, narrowly averted meltdown at the Three Mile Island nuclear power plant in 1979, the nuclear threat that created the climate of the Cold War made the idea of putting radioactive material in the body wildly unpopular.

Still, some good came out of the research. Experiments done in Houston on the effects of radiation in animals showed that the body could tolerate more than was initially believed. Over a period of four or so years, technicians implanted plutonium capsules in the abdomens of dogs and baboons, and from 1975 to 1977, twenty-one humans wore plutonium-powered pacemakers outside their bodies to determine what kinds of problems, if any, the radioactive material caused. The answer was: not much, unless you counted setting off alarms in metal detectors.

By the 1980s, nuclear medicine was, in fact, a growing specialty, with new radiopharmaceuticals used for diagnosing everything from heart and kidney disease to tear duct blockages. PET scanners used in imaging and diagnosis make use of a dye with radioactive tracers.

It may be that the need for a nuclear-powered battery for an artificial heart has already been eclipsed by newer, less threatening technology. In the early 2000s, a completely implantable pump called the Abiocor was developed by a team headed by a Massachusetts aerospace engineer, David M. Lederman, and a PhD scientist, Robert Kung. To Bud's way of thinking, it was a pretty good device: though pulsatile, the Abiocor had no air compressor and recharged itself wirelessly, sending messages through the skin. The internal battery and a controller that monitored the heart rate sat comfortably near the abdomen.

As usual, the makers came to Bud for implantation. He put it in fourteen patients in FDA-approved clinical trials in 2001; *Time* magazine heralded the Abiocor as its Invention of the Year soon after. The longest-living patient, Tom Christerson, survived for 512 days after receiving the Abiocor in Louisville, Kentucky. The most popular patient was a tall, thin African American named Robert Tools, who became a medical celebrity for a time.

Lederman was optimistic. "There is no reason a person should die when their heart stops," he told CBS News. "If the person's brain and the rest of the body is in good shape, why should people die?"

It was a good question, and the answer in the case of the Abiocor lay, once again, with money and human frailty more than medical progress.

The Abiocor was never powerful enough to serve as a permanent replacement for the heart, because the membranes weren't strong enough. Most patients got about five months of life from its use. The pump was also complex—it had lots of moving parts—and very large, about the size of a grapefruit, so the only people it would fit were very large men. And it came with a $700,000 price tag. Even so, the Abiocor could have been used as a bridge to transplant for a limited population, but Lederman wasn't interested. He couldn't make enough money on a market that small, and the Abiocor vanished from cardiac history, apart from a starring role in a 2009 movie called *Crank: High Voltage.*

In the movie, Jason Statham plays a man whose real heart is removed by Chinese mobsters and replaced with an artificial one, played by the Abiocor. Static electricity is supposed to keep the heart's battery going, so the Statham character tries to keep himself charged at first by rubbing against as many people as possible to create friction, and then by having sex with an amenable stripper. It sounded a lot more appealing than partnering forever with a battery pack.

THE DREAM OF ETERNAL LIFE

The LVAD floor at St. Luke's wasn't what anyone would call a happy place: a lot of the patients were aged and bedbound, barely conscious in darkened rooms. One middle-aged patient was on hiatus from his nursing home, propped up in bed with socks tumbling down his ankles, his mouth wide open in what looked to be a nearly perpetual slumber. Others looked pretty good, chatting with relatives in various languages while they waited for whatever surgery or tune-up they needed. Bud knew a great many of them from years past—he'd operated on them, or consulted on their cases, and the recognition would light up their faces and his.

The people swarming around the dimly lit nursing station were another matter. In 2017, they didn't know Bud and he didn't know them, a situation that had been all too obvious a few nights before, when a woman named Sharon Stone had reached him by phone in his office, trying to get a sick friend from Beaumont, Texas, admitted to St. Luke's.

Bud asked about her friend's history and condition, and about the woman's relationship to the patient. "He was my manager," she told him. Bud asked what business she was in. "You may have seen me in some movies," she said.

Time had not slowed him down much, even if he was closing in on seventy-seven. "Well," Bud said, laying the Texas on thick, "if you are the Sharon Stone I'm thinking about I guess I've seen a lot of you."

The story gave Bud a chuckle over the next few days, but his clever comeback was not the punch line. The punch line was that when he called to check on the patient after finding a cardiologist to admit him in the middle of the night, the nurse on the cardiac floor refused to give him any information because she didn't know who he was. "This actress in Hollywood knows more about me than a nurse in my own hospital," he said, shaking his head.

Indeed, his presence on the LVAD floor had become, literally, academic. Bud had a new job leading rounds once a month for medical students, interns, residents, nurses, surgeons, and anyone else who cared to attend. The diversity of the group today would have been unimaginable when Bud was their age: there were a number of women present, and the number of white men in attendance was decidedly small. Asian, Middle Eastern, African, and African American—they all listened with varying degrees of attention. Most of them weren't yet alive when Robert Jarvik put a heart in Barney Clark—"Jarvik was a great machinist but he didn't know anything about medicine . . ."—much less when Denton Cooley stole the heart from his nemesis Michael DeBakey, and they probably didn't care.

LVADs, like any number of former medical miracles, had gone the way of the space shuttle; the glamour and drama of open-heart surgery was gone. Much surgery now could be done with small incisions and even smaller scopes and tools. No one had to come to the Texas Medical Center to get an LVAD; any good city hospital had a specialist who could put one in. Even so, it was a point of pride with Bud that the work had started here and that, as he often said of the continuous-flow devices and told the students now, "not one had pumped to failure." The machines outlived their human hosts. Maybe the pumps couldn't restore a sick person to his or her previous, active life—patients were still attached to hoses and batteries and countless medications—but they lived, which to many was enough.

Bud's own life had become significantly restricted in the last few months as well, and not just because of his health. Over the decades, both the hospital and Baylor had tried to rein in Bud's save-everyone-and-damn-the-costs tendencies. In this increasingly litigious, prohibitively expensive, and data-driven age, Bud's willingness to take big risks for those with the least chance of survival was no longer viewed as a plus. He could exhaust the blood bank with complex surgeries; if his patients had no insurance, the hospital had to eat the bills, including their extensive hospital stays. And, again, there were the numbers: Whenever Bud operated on the sickest of the sick—the least likely to survive—he endangered the hospital's mortality statistics, which were becoming ever more crucial for federal reimbursements. (His success rates with patients who were not so close to death were excellent.)

The times caught up with him, not just economically but physically. Depending on who you ask, Bud either asked to operate less because of his back or his knees, or the hospital tried to ease him out of the operating room. Baylor brought in a much younger man from the Northeast who was supposed to take control; at least he now had most of the titles Bud had always been so proud of. He was a small, pale New Yorker who had trained, among other places, at the prestigious Columbia Presbyterian. He also wore a yarmulke—far from normal headwear in the med center, even in 2015—and was exceedingly deferential to Bud, treading lightly, as if he were almost embarrassed to be nearby. It didn't work; it was like sending in the waterboy to give instructions to the star quarterback.

But Bud was more and more alone. He lost Cooley near the end of 2016, in November. Bud's mentor had slipped into a depression after his wife of seventy years had died the month before, and though Cooley had been frail for a number of years, at ninety-six he had quickly grown frailer, his voice softer and his blue eyes rimmed in red. Still, Cooley continued to show up at his office every day, just as he had for decades, though now his hours were shorter. Bud made a point of stopping in regularly, sometimes just to trade a story both had heard a thousand times before, or to complain about the latest indignity by some bean-counting hospital administrator. Cooley, in fact, still had an appetite for any bad news having to do with Methodist Hospital. But then he missed one day at the office and then another, and then he was gone.

The memorial service was held at his family church, a massive stone structure with soaring ceilings lit with glorious stained-glass windows, one of which was in honor of the daughter Cooley had lost to suicide. Bud came in with Rachel just before the service started and looked around in confusion, as if trying to find his usual seat next to the man he had loved for so long.

Billy left in the spring, moving into a new office in an old Nabisco cookie factory that had been repurposed to house the spanking-new Johnson & Johnson Center for Device Innovation. The problems and politics at THI/CHI had infuriated him, particularly when some administrators and board members asked why they shouldn't have a piece of present and future inventions. This was a new era; in Cooley's day no one would have dared to suggest such a thing. Billy's new gig seemed like a good one, though he worried that people would lose respect for him because he wasn't doing much heart surgery and, at the same time, that J&J would have issues with his eccentricities. But meeting and greeting corporate types fit his personality pretty well—it wasn't so different from performing magic tricks—as did hosting seminars for would-be inventors and entrepreneurs. They hoped that his advice or potential influence could land them the chance to develop and sell their product or their company to Johnson & Johnson. At one event, he was cornered by not one but two people who had invented what they believed were better, more user-friendly tests for stool samples. ("No shit!" Billy responded, meeting them.)

If Bud, Billy, and Daniel were still a ways from putting the Bivacor in a person, they had to be ready, just in case the emergency opportunity arose, as it had with Craig Lewis. They often met at MITIE, Methodist Hospital's Institute for Technology, Innovation, and Education, which had the best morgue in the med center, a sun-washed room on a high floor of yet another new building. It looked more like a state-of-the-art spacecraft than the grim, dank morgues of television detective stories.

Calf studies told them a lot, but in order to save a person, they had to know how the device would best fit in a human body. Hence their presence in the morgue. They wore scrubs but no masks or caps—this wasn't a sterile atmosphere. The corpse was laid out on a table, barely visible under a light blue paper sheet that slipped and revealed various parts of the body as Billy and Daniel hovered over and around the chest cavity. This was someone who had lived a good long time. His skin had the pinkish-gray pallor of the dead kept in cold storage, and he looked to have been a big man in life. His mottled, shaved head was massive, as were his thighs, which happened to be the spot where his legs ended, the skin tucked back in on itself where his knees should have been. His stubby fingers peeked out from beneath the drape whenever someone brushed against it;

occasionally his penis and scrotum appeared as a furry, listless heap. Maybe he had been a bank president, or maybe he had been a greeter at Walmart; in this state all anyone could discern was that he had been generous enough to let a couple of guys use what he left behind for medical research.

They opened the chest with a quick flick of the scalpel and spread the layers of muscle aside. Daniel put the Bivacor in, feeling around for familiar guideposts, shifting and shoving it this way and that, looking for the way the machine would or might better connect to various parts of the body. Long ago, Jarvik had insisted that the only way an artificial heart would be successful was if the person hosting it could forget that it was there. Hence this exercise. How deep should it go? What was the best, most precise angle to connect to the body? Should they change the angles of the tubes protruding from the device to better direct the flow of blood?

They took measurements, calling out numbers to an assistant who recorded them on a yellow pad. It wasn't so different from buying a custom suit, and in some future, maybe closer than Bud's grandfather would want to imagine, the artificial heart would be made that way: programmed to size before it was even manufactured, a perfect fit, just like the custom-made cowboy boots Billy and Bud wore as a tribute to a lost, limitless world.

The calf experiments continued too, as the team moved closer to formal FDA trials. Jim and Linda came occasionally to watch, as did surgeons Bud had worked with over the years. Former patients came too.

One of those was Ally Babineaux, twenty-nine. Her trouble had started in 2008 when Ally, a fierce college athlete, collapsed after a rowing contest. She got a diagnosis of strep throat at her college medical center, but instead of bouncing back like she always did, Ally got sicker and weaker. She went to several more doctors, but no one could tell her what was wrong—she just kept fainting. Maybe she was working out too hard, one doctor suggested. Maybe she was dehydrated. Maybe it was her gallbladder.

More time passed, and was lost, before Ally's parents insisted on taking her to St. Luke's, where doctors finally diagnosed her with viral cardiomyopathy, a disease of the heart muscle that can be fatal. She was in the prime of her life: a beautiful Texas blonde with flashing brown eyes and the toughness of a pit bull. Ally was also engaged to be married at the time; suddenly she wasn't sure whether she should be planning her wedding or her funeral. Finally her cardiologist laid out the best options for survival: a transplant or an assist device. The transplant waiting list numbered in the thousands, and besides, Ally didn't want one. A pump could come out when she was better, she thought, and she would be whole again.

That was when she met her surgeon, Bud Frazier, an odd duck who used nothing more than his hands to measure how and where he was going to cut and where he was going to place something called the HeartMate II inside her body. Maybe because Ally was the same age and had the same name as his daughter, or maybe because she was such a fighter, arguing with her healthcare team, or maybe for all those reasons, Ally became one of Bud's favorites. He checked on her at all hours, and answered her (sometimes angry) phone calls, and would rush to her room when she became agitated or delusional. But she survived, marrying at twenty, a vision in a lacy white gown, with Bud watching quietly from a back row. *People* magazine wrote a story, christening Ally the "Bionic Bride."

But a year or so later, her health began to fail again, just months after she had begun to feel strong enough to consider taking her pump out. This time no machine could save her, because too much of her heart was damaged. Her only hope was a transplant. Ally moved back into St. Luke's as first her kidneys and then her liver shut down. She spent months in the hospital just waiting, too sick to leave, battling depression, sometimes on a respirator, off and on dialysis. No one was sure she would survive. But she did, walking out of the hospital with a new heart in 2011. Ally had to have a second transplant in 2014 after the first resulted in a case of arterial sclerosis—the arteries in her new heart began to clog, something that sometimes happens to young female patients. That hospital stay lasted 178 days.

One day, while Ally was still recovering in the hospital, Bud asked her to meet him in his conference room. She thought that her temper might have landed her in trouble again, maybe for snapping at a nurse.

Instead, Bud sat her down and began to tell her a story. It was about a young Italian boy he'd tried to save as an intern; he'd been fine, and then had gone into heart failure. Bud had squeezed his heart to keep it beating, but for nothing. He'd had to let him go. Just when Ally was beginning to wonder why Bud was telling her this particular story, she understood. Her heart had stopped beating too, and Bud had reached deep into her chest and squeezed and squeezed until he forced her back to life. Unlike the boy who haunted Bud's dreams, Ally had made it.

Now here she was, with her mother, Krista, watching intently as Bud, Billy, Daniel, and a whole crew in sky-blue scrubs sewed a tiny mechanical heart inside a sacrificial calf so that maybe one day the same machine might save someone who was desperate for more time, no matter how short or how long, no matter the cost or the pain.

They wandered outside the operating room and into the Bivacor lair, where one of the techs showed them the glass case with all the artificial hearts that had led to this one. Krista gave her daughter a long look that was hopeful and helpless in equal parts. She hitched a thumb in the direction of the OR. "You'd better hurry up," she said, "so that thing's ready when Ally needs it."

Bud didn't hear her. He was still in surgery, cutting and stitching, still trying to make a heart that wouldn't break.

ACKNOWLEDGMENTS

At about the same time I signed the contract for this book, my father came to spend the last years of his life with my husband, John, and me. I mention this because caring for him was not just a challenge for the two of us, but for all the people at Crown who went above and beyond in their care and concern for *Ticker* while I was often torn between two eerily linked tasks. Editor Roger Scholl's patience, thoughtfulness, and unflagging enthusiasm for this book kept me going on days when I was racing from the emergency room to my desk and back again. The same is true of his editorial assistant Erin Little—her sunny, supportive presence is rivaled only by her velvet-gloved efficiency.

The entire Crown team's enthusiasm for and loyalty to *Ticker* has just been overwhelming. Publisher Molly Stern and associate publisher Annsley Rosner had my back from the very beginning and never wavered, always providing crucial suggestions to make the book better. Publicist Liz Esman and marketer Becca Putman have been a font of creative ideas and unbridled energy, for which I will be eternally grateful. The brilliance of text designer Songhee Kim and jacket designer Chris Brand left me in awe—Chris designed not one, but two covers that took my breath away. And to Norman Watkins and Cindy Berman, production manager and senior production editor, respectively, I add a thousand apologies for what had to have been inconveniences that would have taxed the most serene of Buddhist monks.

The same is true of my longtime friend and agent David McCormick, whose encouragement and support provided just the right amount of jet fuel to get me started on what was another daunting project, one that turned out to be a lot harder than writing about Enron. Thanks too to Brian Sweany, Jake Silverstein, Tim Taliaferro, and Paul Hobby at *Texas Monthly* for what became a much longer leave of absence than I ever intended.

I was so lucky to have the most overqualified intern in the history of journalism—Emily Schaffer, graduate of Harvard law and budding novelist—who performed the tortures of microfiche and bibliographical research, among other torments, with grace, accuracy, and good humor. Sarah Hartzell was a lifesaver when it came to research in D.C. and taught me the value of Drop Box.

My husband, John, was not only a careful, thoughtful reader, but a constant source of love and the best title inventor on the planet. Dario Robleto not only showed me there was a book in the artificial heart, but spent countless hours in nerdy discussions on, yes, the meaning of it all. Doris Taylor, Emily Yoffe, Jan Jarboe Russell, Meg Boulware, Mary Teague, Andrew Gol, Frank Michel, Ken Hoge, Ruth Sorelle, Susan Cooley, Jane Grande Allen, Claudia Feldman, Richard Wampler, and Mike Friedman shared unique insights that shaped my thinking; a thousand thanks to Jill Jewett, Lisa Belkin, Bruce Gelb, Roberta Ness, and Kate Rodemann for the thankless task of reading a first draft and giving me their honest opinions about what needed to be done. Amy Hertz proved to be an incisive and thoughtful reader as well; it's hard to know what was more valuable, her merciless line edits or her big-picture ideas.

In books, as in stories, there is always one person who ends up as the author's go-to—the person who isn't the subject of the book but who is so knowledgeable and so accomplished that he or she can answer any question from the dumbest to the most arcane. Marianne Mallia was that person for *Ticker*—a brilliant medical writer and editor whose patience as a former high school teacher prepared her for my constant assaults on her workday. This book could not have happened without her.

The same is true of the patients and relatives of patients, and to Robert Jarvik who urged me to talk with them in depth. Thanks a thousand times to Linda Lewis, Joel Karp, Ally Babineaux, Tara Templeton, and her extremely perceptive daughter, Shana. My deepest gratitude for your willingness to share such powerful memories, and my apologies for the pain this must have caused.

Billy Cohn, Mishaun Cohn, Daniel Timms, Mack and Linda McIngvale, and so many others at the Texas Heart Institute were dragged into this project unwittingly as it grew ever larger. Their patience with someone whose technical knowledge initially extended to *The Heart/The Kid's Question & Answer Book* will never be forgotten, nor will my gratitude—thanks for allowing me to interrupt work that was always far more important than mine.

To Rachel, Todd, and Allison Frazier, thank you so much for sharing your husband and father with me, for digging into closets for nearly lost CDs, and for excavating your memories; ditto Libby Schwenke, who I wish could organize my life as well as she organizes her boss's every day. To Bud Frazier, who must have never imagined I would actually finish: well, thanks for sharing a life of amazing riches and challenges, and for not once losing patience when I asked for the thousandth time to explain the compliance chamber. I know you signed on to this without a clue as to what you were getting into, and the kindness, doggedness, and graciousness you extended to me was the same as that you give to your patients, who love you for it still. You never gave up, and, I know, never will.

NOTES

PROLOGUE

The bulk of this chapter is drawn from personal interviews with Linda Lewis, Bud Frazier, and Frank Michel.

CHAPTER 1: THE WIZARD, 2015

The bulk of this chapter was drawn from personal interviews with Bud Frazier, Frank Michel, Betsy Parish, Denton Cooley, and others who recalled the boom days of the Texas Medical Center. Some of it is also drawn from personal recollection.

17 He had told his mother: Paul Harasim, "O. H. 'Bud' Frazier, M.D.," *Innovator,* St. Luke's Episcopal Hospital Magazine, Winter 2001/2002, 7.

18 a total replacement that could be implanted: Harold M. Schmeck Jr., "Artificial Heart Research Now Seeks a Portable and 'Forgettable' Device," *New York Times,* December 6, 1982.

CHAPTER 2: HOW HARD COULD IT BE?

Personal interviews include Bud Frazier, Betsy Parish, Marianne Mallia, and others, including patients and friends with heart disease. The facts and figures on heart disease come mainly from the American Heart Association, https://www .heart.org/idc/groups/ahamah-public/@wcm/@sop/@smd/documents/down loadable/ucm_480086.pdf, and various other sources on heart disease. I read many books on the history of the heart, cardiology, and heart disease, which are listed in the bibliography. I did find this book to be one of the best: Stephen Amidon and Thomas Amidon, *The Sublime Engine: A Biography of the Human*

Heart (Emmaus, PA: Rodale Books, 2012). On the availability of donor hearts, there are also many sources, but one is http://www.syncardia.com/total-facts /donor-heart-facts.html. On the rise in heart failure and the decline of heart attacks, see, among other stories, Gina Kolata, "For Patients with Heart Failure, Little Guidance as Death Nears," *New York Times*, November 6, 2017.

23 Many modern-day inventors: My interview with Richard Wampler was particularly helpful.

24 To explore the workings of the heart: Again, my description of heart function comes from a compilation of several books and websites. I confess to resorting to several from the Khan Academy, which were very helpful. See, for instance, Khan Academy, "Heart Disease and Heart Attacks," https://www.youtube .com/watch?v=_wre2WRPiFI, and the information on Armando Hasundungan's website, http://armandoh.org/subjects/cardiology.

27 As late as 1900: James E. Dalen et al., "The Epidemic of the 20th Century: Coronary Heart Disease," *American Journal of Medicine* 127, no. 9 (September 2014): 807–12.

27 Then, on September 24, 1955: Clarence G. Lasby, *Eisenhower's Heart Attack: How Ike Beat Heart Disease and Held On to the Presidency* (Lawrence: University Press of Kansas, 1997); Cody White, *Heart Attack Strikes Ike*, from the National Archives Text Message Blog, September 22, 2016, https://text-message .blogs.archives.gov/2016/09/22/heart-attack-strikes-ike-president-eisenhowers -1955-medical-emergency-in-colorado.

CHAPTER 3: THE MAKING OF A SURGEON

Personal interviews with Bud Frazier, Denton Cooley, Marian Mallia, William Butler, Stephen Igo, and Claudia Feldman, among others. Much of the history is compiled from multiple sources, as well as having grown up in Texas myself. Bud Frazier is the best source on his own history, but the story by Paul Harasim cited above, as well as a few mentioned below, was particularly helpful. As for the history of heart surgery, I used the Albion brothers' book along with several others listed in the bibliography.

31 Despite that, Bryant ran: Jim Dent, *The Junction Boys: How Ten Days in Hell with Bear Bryant Forged a Championship Team* (New York; St. Martin's Press, 2000).

34 Michael DeBakey had landed: For DeBakey's beginnings in Houston, I relied on many sources, but among the best was William T. Butler and Diane L. Ware, *Arming for Battle Against Disease Through Education, Research and Patient Care at Baylor College of Medicine* (Houston, TX: Baylor College of Medicine, 2011). Much of the book was helpful, but in particular pages 37–42. I also drew on: *Houston Hearts: A History of Cardiovascular Surgery and Medicine*

and the Methodist DeBakey Heart and Vascular Center (Elisha Freeman Publishing, Houston, 2014); Kenneth L. Mattox, *The History of Surgery in Houston: Fifty-Year Anniversary of the Houston Surgical Society* (Austin, TX: Eakin Press, 1998).

35 He was nothing if not focused: Mimi Swartz, "Till Death Do Us Part," *Texas Monthly*, March 2005; NIH, US National Library of Medicine, The Michael E. DeBakey Papers, from Tulane School of Medicine to the US Army, 1928–1946; Thomas Thompson; "A Bitter Feud," *Life*, April 10, 1970, 8; Winters, *Houston Hearts*, chs. 1, 3, 4. Also see the Michael DeBakey Papers, US National Library of Medicine, https://profiles.nim.nih.gov/ps/retrieve/Narrative/FJ/p-nid/322.

36 It was there that some of: John E. Salvaggio, *New Orleans' Charity Hospital: A Story of Physicians, Politics, and Poverty* (Baton Rouge: Louisiana State University Press, 1992), 147.

37 Baylor, he wrote, was: Butler, Butler and Ware, *Arming for Battle*, 37–42.

38 That was never truer than: John F. Kennedy Moon Speech, https://er.jsc.nasa.gov/seh/ricetalk.htm.

40 Winning the Lasker Prize was not: Elizabeth Drew, "The Health Syndicate: Washington's Noble Conspirators," *Atlantic Monthly*, December 1967, 75–82.

43 DeBakey also found a way: There are many accounts of this story, but I trusted Butler's account in *Arming for Battle*, as he was a close friend of DeBakey's, as well as supporting documents from his own papers, https://profiles.nlm.nih.gov/ps/retrieve/Narrative/FJ/p-nid/322.

44 "We are on the brink": Michael DeBakey, speech to Congress, US Congress, Senate Subcommittee of the Committee on Appropriations for 1963 Hearings on Department of Health, Education, and Welfare Appropriations (Washington, DC: GPO, 1963), 1402.

CHAPTER 4: A TOUR OF HELL

Even though Bud plays down his Vietnam service, I did make use of his video compilation and the recorded letters he sent home, as well as notebooks Bud kept at the time. I also interviewed several other combat veterans, most notably Michael Freedman, whose help was invaluable. For historical context, I drew particularly on Ken Burns' ten-part series on the Vietnam War. Other interviewees for the section on DeBakey included his longtime associate George Noon. On Cooley's skills, I interviewed Bud Frazier and many other medical associates.

52 Bud was drafted as part of the Berry Plan: Frank B. Berry, "The Story of the 'Berry Plan,'" *Bulletin of the New York Academy of Medicine* 52, no. 3 (March–April 1976): 278–82.

52 One of his closest friends: Bill Bramer, "Salvation Worries? Prostate Trouble?," *Texas Monthly*, March 1973.

55 The dense, triple-canopy mountains: James T. Gillam, *Life and Death in the Central Highlands: An American Sergeant in the Vietnam War, 1968–1970*, North Texas Military Biography and Memoir Series (Denton, TX: University of North Texas Press, 2010), 13, 79, 84, 115.

57 "Be like a rocky promontory": Marcus Aurelius Antonius, *Meditations*, trans. George Long (Sioux Falls, SD: Nu Vision Publications, 2008), 32.

58 "I got a vitamin deficiency": Tommy Thompson, *Hearts* (London: Pan Books, 1974), 244.

58 Bud found himself drawn to the neighboring Texas Heart Institute: *Twenty-Five Years of Excellence: A History of the Texas Heart Institute* (Houston: Texas Heart Institute Foundation, 1989), 10–19.

CHAPTER 5: THE WAR AT HOME

Interviews with Denton Cooley, Bud Frazier, Denis DeBakey, George Noon, and Ruth Sylvester, among others. Cooley's history comes from personal interviews, as well as three books: Tommy Thompson's *Hearts*; Harry Minetree's *Cooley: The Amazing Career of the World's Greatest Surgeon* (New York: Harper's Magazine Press, 1973); and Denton Cooley's autobiography, *100,000 Hearts: A Surgeon's Memoir* (Austin: Dolph Briscoe Center for American History, University of Texas, 2012).

62 That predilection had to have come: Ibid., chs. 2–3.

64 Still, his life wasn't trouble-free: Ibid., 24–25.

65 Once there, he became a favorite: Ibid., ch. 5, for a summary of the Blalock years, including the "blue baby" surgery. Also see Minetree, *Cooley*, ch. 7.

67 Even for a native Houstonian: Jan de Hartog (New York: Atheneum, 1964).

67 The halls were crowded: J. R. Gonzales, "Busy Days, Busy Nights at Jefferson Davis Hospital," *Bayou City History* blog, *Houston Chronicle*, March 14, 2012, http://blog.chron.com/bayoucityhistory/2012/03/busy-days-busy-nights-at-jefferson-davis-hospital.

68 On Cooley's first day: Cooley, *100,000 Hearts*, 90.

70 DeBakey published a paper: Minetree, *Cooley*, 127.

71 "I'm often obliged": David Monagan with David O. Williams, *Journey into the Heart: A Tale of Pioneering Doctors and Their Race to Transform Cardiovascular Medicine* (New York: Gotham Books, 2007).

71 Heart surgery in its: The history of the heart-lung machine and Cooley's use of it comes from multiple sources, including Cooley's autobiography as well as several other histories, including Amidon and Amidon, *The Sublime Engine*,

and G. Wayne Miller, *King of Hearts: The True Story of the Maverick Who Pioneered Open Heart Surgery* (New York: Times Books, 2000).

72 Yeager, however, was never prosecuted: G. Wayne Miller, *King of Hearts, The True Story of the Maverick Who Pioneered Heart Surgery* (New York: Crown Publishers, 2000), 227–240.

74 DeBakey had kept close tabs on Cooley's progress: Cooley, *100,000 Hearts*, 105.

75 Mary Lasker wrote of: Mary Lasker, Columbia University Libraries Oral History Research Office, Notable New Yorkers, Part 1, Session 36, 1110.

75 He populated his formal office: Minetree, *Cooley*, 185.

76 The brilliant surgeon Adrian Kantrowitz: My account of the global race to transplant a heart comes from several books and news articles, including Cooley, *100,000 Hearts*; Thompson, *Hearts*; and David K. C. Cooper, M.D., *Open Heart: The Radical Surgeons Who Revolutionized Medicine* (New York: Kaplan Publishing, 2010).

76 The dog, named Ruff: Adrian Kantrowitz Papers, https://profiles.nlm.nih.gov /ps/retrieve/ResourceMetadata/GNBBKL.

77 On this point, Kantrowitz: *NOVA: The Artificial Heart*, PBS, aired October 18, 1983.

77 The legal and medical definition of death: Several sources were used in the brief account of brain death definition, including Calixto Machado et al., "The Concept of Brain Death Did Not Evolve to Benefit Organ Transplants," *Journal of Medical Ethics* 33, no. 4 (April 2007): 197–200; as well as Michael A. De Georgia, "History of Brain Death as Death: 1968 to the Present," *Journal of Critical Care* 29, no. 4 (August 2014): 673–78.

77 He distracted himself: Many sources were used in the account of the beginnings of the Texas Heart Institute, including Cooley's autobiography and the Texas Heart Institute Foundation's *Twenty-Five Years of Excellence.*

78 "The pump was still working": Domingo Liotta, *Amazing Adventures of a Heart Surgeon: The Artificial Heart: The Frontiers of Human Life* (Lincoln, NE: iUniverse, 2007), 173.

78 DeBakey also used federal grants: William Akers, interview, along with various news clippings on the Rice/Baylor collaboration.

78 Rice engineers were then known: Michael E. DeBakey, "The Odyssey of the Artificial Heart," *Artificial Organs* vol 24, no. 6 (2000): 405–11.

79 Then, in August 1966: Many accounts exist of the Esperanza del Valle Vasquez procedure. Sources here included Winters, *Houston Hearts*; DeBakey, "Odyssey of the Artificial Heart."

CHAPTER 6: THE PURLOINED HEART

The account of the growing feud between Cooley and DeBakey and the implantation of the artificial heart in Haskell Karp comes from multiple sources, including *Life* magazine, "The Feud," the *New York Times*, Cooley's autobiography, Domingo Liotta's autobiography, Tommy Thompson's *Hearts*, and DeBakey, "Odyssey of the Artificial Heart." I am also extremely grateful to the family of Haskell and Miriam Karp for allowing me to read Mrs. Karp's diary of that difficult time. Interviews also include those with Cooley, Frazier, et cetera. I am also deeply indebted to Renee C. Fox and Judith P. Swazey, whose account of the implantation in chapter 6 of *The Courage to Fail: A Social View of Organ Transplants and Dialysis* (New Brunswick, NJ: Transaction, 2013) is truly outstanding.

84 "Congratulations on your first transplant": Cooley, *100,000 Hearts*, 125.

85 "Maybe it's immodest of me": Cooley, Ibid., 125.

85 "Denton just got tired of sucking hind tit": Thomas Thompson, "The Texas Tornado vs. Dr. Wonderful," *Life*, April 10, 1970, 69.

88 Other surgeons around the world were reporting: Thomas Thompson, "The Year They Changed Hearts: A New and Disquieting Look at Transplants," *Life*, September 17, 1971, 56–70.

88 Many in the press thought: Judith Randal, "Transplants, Apollo Both Misguided?" *Washington Star*, January 26, 1969.

88 "I can respect": Denton Cooley, *Essays of Denton A. Cooley, M.D.: Reflections and Observations* (Austin, TX: Eakin Press, 1984).

90 Then, on a sweltering day in July: Cooley, *100,000 Hearts*, 89–90.

93 "Cooley and I moved forward": Liotta, *Amazing Adventures of a Heart Surgeon*, 194.

96 "Domingo, we administered": Ibid., 199.

CHAPTER 7: EXPERIMENTS

Interviewees for this chapter include Marianne Mallia, Bud Frazier, Steve Parnis, Betsy Parish, Ruth SoRelle, Ruth Sylvester, Michael Jhin, and others.

98 DeBakey had learned: Statement of Dr. Michael E. DeBakey, made to the executive committee of the Baylor College of Medicine Board of Trustees, April 10, 1969.

99 "A successful cardiovascular surgeon": Stephen Westaby, *Open Heart: A Cardiac Surgeon's Stories of Life and Death on the Operating Table* (New York: Basic Books, 2017).

100 By the early 1970s: Cooley, *100,000 Hearts*, 152–54; also interviews with those mentioned above.

106 One of those was a product: Karl Heusler and Alfred Pletsher, "The Controversial Early History of Cyclosporine," *Swiss Medical Weekly*, June 2, 2001, 21–22, 299–302.

109 Small, intense, and bespectacled: For a good account of Vic Poirier's many contributions, see ASAIO Pioneer Interviews, https://asaio.com/about-us/asaio -pioneer-interviews. See also Jonathan B. Welch, "Case Study: Heart, Soul and Cash at Thermo Cardiosystems, Inc.," *Journal of Financial Education* 29 (Winter 2003): 90–112.

111 Eventually Frazier, working with Cooley and Norman: O. H. Frazier, "Mechanical Cardiac Assistance: Historical Perspectives," *Seminars in Thoracic and Cardiovascular Surgery* 12, no. 3 (July 2000): 207–20. See also O. H. Frazier, "Mechanical Circulatory Assist Device Development at the Texas Heart Institute: A Personal Perspective," *Seminars in Thoracic and Cardiovascular Surgery* 26, no. 1 (Spring 2014): 4–13.

CHAPTER 8: BARNEY WHO?

Many interviews and much research went into this chapter, including, of course, Bud Frazier and Robert Jarvik. Once again, outstanding work on this episode in American medical history was done by Fox and Swazey in *Spare Parts*. Also see Margery Shaw, ed., *After Barney Clark: Reflections on the Utah Artificial Heart Program* (Austin: University of Texas Press, 1984). Great work was also done by the Canadian medical historian Shelley McKellar in "Limitations Exposed: Willem J. Kolff and His Contentious Pursuit of a Mechanical Heart," in *Essays in Honour of Michael Bliss: Figuring the Social*, ed. E. A. Heaman, Alison Li, and Shelley McKellar (Toronto: University of Toronto Press, 2008). Also see Barron H. Lerner, *When Illness Goes Public: Celebrity Patients and How We Look at Medicine* (Baltimore: Johns Hopkins University Press, 2006), 180–200.

118 "The Artificial Heart Is Here": James Salter and Marie Claude Wren, "The Artificial Heart Is Here," *Life*, September 1981, 28–36.

118 As far as the general public knew: Several accounts of DeBakey's revenge exist, including Cooley's in *100,000 Hearts*, 144–48. I also completed an interview with Al Rienert, whose lively account of the trial appeared in the *Houston Chronicle* in June 1972. There also exists a video dramatization of the legal proceedings entitled "The Trial of Denton Cooley," *NOVA*, PBS Television, 1978.

120 "should have stimulated further clinical trials": Cooley, *Essays of Denton A. Cooley*, 104.

121 When he ran into Akutsu: Salter and Wren, "Artificial Heart Is Here," 31–36.

126 For the last few months: My account of the Barney Clark surgery comes largely from the sources cited above, as well as Salter and Wren, "Artificial Heart Is Here."

126 "the body as an entity of replaceable parts": Alison Li, et al. (eds.), *Limitations Exposed: Willem S. Kolff and His Contentious Pursuit of a Mechanical Heart* (Toronto: University of Toronto Press, 2008), 400.

129 He cast his net so widely: Nicholas Genes, "Paul Winchell and the Artificial Heart," MedGadget, July 1, 2005, https://www.medgadget.com/2005/07 /paul_winchell_a.html. To view his US patent no. 3097366, see https://www .google.com/patents/US3097366.

129 At Kolff's direction: Janny Scott, "Lack of Recognition Embitters Some Pioneers of Artificial Heart Design," *Los Angeles Times*, January 4, 1987.

130 In a classic example: Robert Jarvik, "The Total Artificial Heart," *Scientific American*, January 1981, 74.

131 It must have galled the Utah surgeons: Cooley, *Essays of Denton A. Cooley*, 139.

132 As a headline in *People* put it: Frank W. Martin, "Utah Surgeon William DeVries Seeks a Patient Who Could Live with a Man-Made Heart," *People*, July 19, 1982, 30–31.

133 Clark was, in short, a brave: The fascinating psychological report that is threaded through this chapter is cited as follows: Claudia K. Berenson and Bernard I. Grosser, "Total Artificial Heart Implantation," *Archives of General Psychiatry* 41 (September 1984): 910–16.

137 Their authority would be questioned: President's Commission for the Study of Ethical Problems in Medicine and Biomedical and Behavioral Research, *Congressional Record*, October 14, 1978; "The President's Commission for the Study of Ethical Problems in Medicine and Biomedical and Behavioral Research: A Guide to the Records in the Bioethics Research Library," Kennedy Institute of Ethics, Georgetown University, Washington, DC, https:// bioethics.georgetown.edu/archives/Presidents-Commission-for-Study-of -Ethical-Problems-in-Medicine-and-in-Biomedical-and-Behavioral-Research -Original-Archive-Finding-Aid.pdf.

137 Not coincidentally: As stated above, much of this account draws on the work of Fox and Swazey, *Spare Parts*.

138 That eleven-page consent form: Shaw, ed., *After Barney Clark*, Appendix A.

138 But it was Barton J. Bernstein: Barton J. Bernstein, "The Misguided Quest for the Artificial Heart," *Technology Review*, November/December 1984, 19.

CHAPTER 9: THE PRISONER

Interviewees for this chapter included Bud Frazier, Claudia Feldman, and Shana Templeton and her mother, Tara.

141 A government study released in May 1982: Deborah P. Lubeck and John P. Bunker, *The Implications of Cost-Effectiveness Analysis of Medical Technology*,

Background Paper #2: Case Studies of Medical Technologies, Case Study #9: The Artificial Heart: Cost, Risks, and Benefits (Washington, DC: GPO, 1982).

142 Over time, with more experiments: Thermo Cardiosystems Inc., "HeartMate Left Ventricular-Assist System," October 1995.

142 Mike Templeton was a very young: The accounts of Mike Templeton's life come from multiple interviews but also the following print accounts of the time: Judith Anne Yeaple, "The Bionic Heart," *Popular Science*, April 1992, 64–69; D. J. Wilson, "Portable Heart Assist Pump Working Fine; Gives Patient Here a Month of New Life," *Houston Chronicle*, October 2, 1991, A-6; Claudia Feldman, "Mike Templeton's Broken Heart: A New Device Keeps His Heart Beating Just Fine, but Now He Wants to Go Home," *Houston Chronicle*, April 12, 1992, A-6; Claudia Feldman, "Then & Now/1991: Mike Templeton," *Houston Chronicle*, July 10, 1994, 15; Michael J. Neill, "Cardiac Arrest," *People*, September 14, 1992; "Man with Experimental Heart Device Dies," *New York Times*, January 21, 1993.

CHAPTER 10: THE WILDERNESS

Interviews: Bud Frazier, Richard Wampler, Steve Parnis, Bob Benkowski, and Marianne Mallia.

147 Since the late 1980s: Among others, "Special Report: The Political History of the Artificial Heart," *New England Journal of Medicine*, February 2, 1984; Ralph Brauer, "The Promise That Failed," *New York Times Magazine*, August 28, 1988; Thomas Preston, "The Artificial Heart," in Diana B. Dutton with contributions by Thomas A. Preston and Nancy E. Pfund, *Worse Than the Disease* (Cambridge: Cambridge University Press, 1988); Gideon Gil, "The Artificial Heart Juggernaut," *Hastings Center Report*, March 1, 1989; Charles Siebert, "The Rehumanization of the Heart: What Doctors Have Forgotten, Poets Have Always Known," *Harper's*, February 1990, 53; Howard Witt, "Soul-Searching over Artificial Hearts Intensifies," *Chicago Tribune*, August 10, 1986.

147 So too did the so-called Baby Fae case: Lawrence K. Altman, "Baby Fae, Who Received a Heart from Baboon, Dies After 20 Days," *New York Times*, November 16, 1984.

148 Much closer to home: Steve McVicker, "Bursting the Bubble," *Houston Press*, April 10, 1997.

148 Then there was the issue of cost: Barton J. Bernstein, "The Artificial Heart: Is It a Boon or a High-Tech Fix?," *The Nation*, June 22, 1983, 71–72.

151 "I was like Robinson Crusoe": Dan Baum, "No Pulse: How Doctors Reinvented the Human Heart," *Popular Science*, March 2012, 4.

152 But after being widowed: "For Dr. DeBakey and His Bride, It Was All Hearts and Flowers," *People* magazine, August 25, 1975.

152 Moreover, it became clear that: Along with interviews, I drew on several accounts of the artificial heart crisis of this period: Brauer, "Promise That Failed"; Philip M. Boffey, "Washington Talk: National Institutes of Health; Battling Congress over Priorities on Heart," *New York Times*, July 8, 1988; Joseph Paul Martino, *Science Funding: Politics and Porkbarrel* (New Brunswick, NJ: Transaction Publishers, 1992), 94–95; "The Dracula of Medical Technology," editorial, *New York Times*, May 16, 1988; "Senators Doctors Kennedy and Hatch," editorial, *New York Times*, July 15, 1988; Robert Jarvik, "Revive Artificial Heart with Money and Vision," letter to the editor, *New York Times*, August 8, 1988; "Claude Lenfant to Retire from National Heart, Lung, and Blood Institute," press release, NHLBI, June 3, 2003.

153 Something else happened: A good general description of the *Challenger* explosion can be found in Diane Vaughan, *The Challenger Launch Decision, Risky Technology, Culture, and Deviance at NASA* (Chicago: University of Chicago Press, 1996). Also Allan J. McDonald, *Truth, Lies and O-Rings: Inside the Space Shuttle* Challenger *Disaster* (Gainesville: University Press of Florida, 2012); Daniel Riffe and James Glen Stovall, "Diffusion of News of Space Shuttle Disaster: What Role for Emotional Response?," *Journalism and Mass Communication Quarterly* 66, no. 3 (September 1989): 551–56; John C. Wright, Dale Kunkel, Marites Pinon, and Aletha C. Houston, "How Children Reacted to Televised Coverage of the Space Shuttle Disaster," *Journal of Communication* 39, no. 2 (June 1, 1989): 27.

156 Like Denton Cooley: Author interviews, Richard Wampler, Bud Frazier, Marianne Mallia; Lawrence K. Altman, "A Tiny Heart Pump Saves Its First Life, Researchers Report," *New York Times*, May 5, 1988; Baum, "No Pulse"; O. E. Frazier, "Mechanical Circulatory Assist Device Development at the Texas Heart Institute: A Personal Perspective," *Journal of Thoracic and Cardiovascular Surgery* 147, no. 6 (June 2014): 1738–44; Steven Phillips, "Project Bionics Pioneer Interview: ASAIO Interviews of Richard Wampler and O. H. Frazier," June 9, 2011, https://asaio.com/about-us/asaio-pioneer-interviews; Richard Wampler, "Tiny, Experimental Pump Offers Hope for Heart Patients," *Los Angeles Times*, August 1, 1988; Richard Wampler, letter to the Awards Committee, Clair Pomeroy Awards, April 4, 2011.

CHAPTER 11: SYNCHRONICITY

Interviewees included Richard Wampler, Robert Jarvik, Marianne Mallia, Bud Frazier, Steve Parnis, and more on background.

165 Bud likes to cite: Michael Walsh, "Change of Hearts: Medical Thriller Provokes Thought," *Reeling Back*, December 3, 2013, http://reelingback.com/articles/change_of_hearts. *Threshold* was written by James Salter, who covered the artificial heart race between Houston and Utah for *Life* magazine in September 1981; http://www.imdb.com/title/tt0083197.

168 The board of the company: Fox and Swazey, *Spare Parts*, 139–40.

169 Having shifted his base of operations: Ibid., 140–47.

169 *Life* magazine's May 1985 story on Schroeder: Jeff Wheelwright, "Bill's Heart: The Troubling Story Behind a Historic Experiment," *Life*, May 1985, 33–42.

170 But, as many celebrities would soon learn: Laurence Gonzales, "The Rock 'n' Roll Heart of Robert Jarvik," *Playboy*, April 1986, 84.

173 By August 1987, Jarvik had divorced: Julie Baumgold, "In the Kingdom of the Brain," *New York Magazine*, February 6, 1989, 36.

175 Jarvik was so upset: Interviews, Bud Frazier, Robert Jarvik, and Marianne Mallia.

175 "I don't know what stage": "Electric Heart," *NOVA*, PBS, aired December 21, 1999, transcript at http://www.pbs.org/wgbh/nova/transcripts/2617eheart.html.

175 If that wasn't bad enough: Baum, "No Pulse." Also Mikhail Iliev, "Absolute Capital Management Leaves Investors Mired in Lawsuits," FINalternatives, April 26, 2011, http://www.finalternatives.com/node/15700.

176 "If you compare it to a prize fight": "Electric Heart," *NOVA*.

CHAPTER 12: THE KING OF DISTRACTION

Interviewees included Billy Cohn, Bud Frazier, Marianne Mallia, Jesse Rios, Mishaun Cohn, Judith Cohn, John Cohn, Bruce Rosengard, Michael Jhin, Betsy Parish, and Ruth SoRelle.

184 "I quickly saw": William Michael Smith, "Rock 'n' Roll Heart," *Oberlin Alumni Magazine*, Winter 2012, http://www2.oberlin.edu/alummag/winter2013/rocknroll.html.

186 The first invention he brought: Jerome Groopman, "Heart Surgery Unplugged: Making the Coronary Bypass Safer, Cheaper, and Easier," *New Yorker*, January 11, 1999, 43.

187 "Like cutting a gemstone": Ibid., 43.

189 He was the old family friend: Todd Ackerman, "Cooley Defends Advice About Cheney," *Houston Chronicle*, October 21, 2013.

193 But this was not to be: Associated Press, "Heart Patient from 'Miracle Workers' Dies," *Today*, March 20, 2006.

CHAPTER 13: HEARTMATES

Interviewees include Bud Frazier, Rich Wampler, Billy Cohn, Bob Benkowski, Ken Hoge, Linda Lewis, Denton Cooley, George Noon, Steve Parnis, Frank Michel, and others on background.

201 As he moved into his eighties: Cooley, *100,000 Hearts*, 193–98.

202 A year or so later, DeBakey nearly died: Lawrence K. Altman, "The Man on the Table Devised the Surgery," *New York Times*, December 25, 2006.

204 "Especially, I am grateful": Cooley, *100,000 Hearts*, 195.

204 And sure enough: Todd Ackerman, "Legendary Heart Surgeons DeBakey, Cooley Mend Rift," *Houston Chronicle*, November 6, 2007.

205 Thousands came to a viewing: Todd Ackerman and Eric Berger, "DeBakey's Death Is a Heartfelt Loss for Houston, World of Medicine," *Houston Chronicle*, July 12, 2008.

206 So on a sunny spring day: Eric Berger, "Artificial Heart 'A Leap Forward,' Houston Docs Say," *Houston Chronicle*, March 23, 2011.

CHAPTER 14: THE AUSTRALIAN GUY

Interviewees include Bud Frazier, Billy Cohn, Daniel Timms, Steve Parnis, and Mariane Mallia. Also, in preparation for a film tribute to Dr. Frazier, a marketing agency called Ttweak conducted extensive interviews with Frazier, Cohn, Timms, and others, from which these scenes are also drawn.

209 Still, the attendant publicity: TEDMED talk with Bud Frazier and Billy Cohn, 2012; Berger, "Artificial Heart 'A Leap Forward.' "

211 To explain how it would work: For those who want more information on the Bivacor and its workings, the website is helpful: www.bivacor.com. Of course, the device has gone through myriad iterations since the scene described here.

216 When Daniel wasn't refining: Most of the biographical information here comes from interviews with Daniel Timms, but I also drew on a few stories from the Australian press, including Trent Dalton, "Bivacor Heart: Daniel Timms' Stroke of Genius," *The Australian*, February 23, 2016.

218 he took his device: Dalton, "Daniel Timms' Stroke of Genius."

CHAPTER 15: MATILDA

Interviewees include Bud Frazier, Billy Cohn, Daniel Timms, Steve Parnis, Denton Cooley, Marianne Mallia, and Jim and Linda McIngvale. Descriptions of the implantations that follow are my own, as I was present.

231 All cities have local celebrities: Biographical information on Jim and Linda McIngvale comes from author interviews and from Jim "Mattress Mack" Mc-

Ingvale with Thomas N. Duening and John M. Ivancevich, *Always Think Big, How Mattress Mack's Uncompromising Attitude Built the Biggest Single Retail Store in America* (Chicago: Dearborn Trade Publishing, 2002).

234 Soon after, without a nap: Eric Berger, "Donor Brings Inventor of Artificial Heart Closer to Houston; Australian Engineer's Device Has Lots of Believers Here," *Houston Chronicle*, January 14, 2013.

CHAPTER 16: THE OCCUPATION

Interviews with Bud Frazier, Billy Cohn, Daniel Timms, Steve Parnis, Jesse Rios, Bruce Rosengard, Jim and Linda McIngvale, and Kerri Sprung.

246 The machine was a success from: Jerome Groopman, "Print Thyself: How 3-D Printing Is Revolutionizing Medicine," *New Yorker*, November 24, 2014.

249 One recent former president: Clifford Pugh, "Former Baylor College of Medicine Prez Peter Traber Marries in a Wacky Las Vegas Ceremony," *Houston Culturemap*, January 2, 2013.

249 He was incensed: "Injecting 420 More Beds into Baylor's Once Catatonic McNair Campus South of the TMC," *Swamplot*, December 21, 2015.

250 But the biggest shock: Todd Ackerman, "St. Luke's Exploring Hospital Sale Options," *Houston Chronicle*, November 3, 2012; Todd Ackerman, "St. Luke's to Sell to National Catholic System," *Houston Chronicle*, April 19, 2013.

251 unveiling the obligatory multimillion-dollar rebranding campaign: Links to the advertising campaigns can be found here: http://tlgadvertising.com/portfolio/living-proof; http://tlgadvertising.com/wp-content/uploads/2015/02/CHISL_CV_NSP_docs1.jpg.

252 There had been a big blowout: Mimi Swartz, "Old Houston Salutes an Irreverent Heart Surgeon," *New York Times*, September 29, 2012.

254 These qualities did not go unnoticed: Mimi Swartz, "It Can't All Be Energy: A Heart Surgeon Leads His City to the Forefront of Medical Innovation," *Texas Monthly*, May 2017.

CHAPTER 17: THE POWER SOURCE

Interviews with Bud Frazier, Billy Cohn, Daniel Timms, Jim and Linda McIngvale, Frank Michel, Robert Jarvik, Allison Balser, and Marianne Mallia.

267 This was not a new idea: Shelley McKellar, "Negotiating Risk: The Failed Development of Atomic Hearts in America, 1967–1977," *Technology and Culture* 54, no. 1 (January 2013).

269 In the early 2000s: Anita Hamilton, "Abiocor Artificial Heart," in "Best Inventions of 2001," *Time*, November 19, 2001.

269 The longest-living patient: Katharine Ristich, "The Last 5 Months of a Fighter: Remembering Robert Tools," *Medscape*, December 3, 2001; John Fisher, "Robert Tools: Artificial Heart Transplant," *To Transplant and Beyond*, http://www.heart-transplant.co.uk/robert.html.

270 "There is no reason a person should die": Dennis Hevesi, "David Lederman, Pioneer of Artificial Heart, Dies at 68," *New York Times*, August 28, 2012.

270 In the movie: For the plot summary, see "Crank: High Voltage," Wikipedia, https://en.wikipedia.org/wiki/Crank:_High_Voltage.

CHAPTER 18: THE DREAM OF ETERNAL LIFE

Interviewees include Bud Frazier, Billy Cohn, and Allison Babineaux.

274 The memorial service was held: "Memorial Service for Denton A. Cooley, MD, November 28, 2016," YouTube, posted by Texas Heart Institute, November 29, 2016, https://www.youtube.com/watch?v=Ugx64djjzbQ.

275 At one event, he was cornered: Swartz, "It Can't All Be Energy."

276 One of those was Ally Babineaux: Alicia Dennis and Darla Atlas, "The Bionic Bride," *People*, June 7, 2010.

277 But a year or so later: Seamus McGraw, "'Bionic Bride' Still in Critical Condition, but 'A Little Better,'" *Today*, January 25, 2011, https://www.today.com /news/bionic-bride-still-critical-condition-little-better-wbna41256873.

SELECTED BIBLIOGRAPHY

BOOKS

Amidon, Stephen, and Thomas Amidon. *The Sublime Engine: A Biography of the Human Heart*. New York: Rodale, 2011.

Bulgakov, Mikhail. *A Country Doctor's Notebook*. London: Harvill Press, 1995.

Butler, William T. *Arming for Battle Against Disease Through Education, Research and Patient Care at Baylor College of Medicine, Book I*. Houston, TX: Baylor College of Medicine, 2011.

Conrad, Peter. *The Sociology of Health and Illness: Critical Perspectives*. New York: Worth, 2009.

Cooley, Denton. *Essays of Denton Cooley, MD: Reflections and Observations*. Austin, TX: Eakin Press, 1973.

Cooley, Denton. *100,000 Hearts: A Surgeon's Memoir*. Austin, TX: Dolph Briscoe Center for American History, University of Texas at Austin, 2012.

Cooper, David K. C. *Open Heart: The Radical Surgeons Who Revolutionized Medicine*. New York: Kaplan, 2010.

DeBakey, Michael E., ed. *The Yearbook of General Surgery*. Chicago: Yearbook Medical, 1970.

Diethrich, Edward B. *SLED: Serendipitous Life of Edward Diethrich*. Wilmington, OH: Orange Frazer Press, 2016.

Dutton, Diana B. *Worse than the Disease: Pitfalls of Medical Progress*. Cambridge: Cambridge University Press, 1988.

Foote, Susan Bartlett. *Managing the Medical Arms Race: Innovation and Public Policy in the Medical Device Industry*. Berkeley: University of California Press, 1992.

Forrester, James S. *The Heart Healers: The Misfits, Mavericks, and Rebels Who Created the Greatest Medical Breakthrough of Our Lives.* New York: St. Martin's Press, 2015.

Fox, Renee C., and Judith P. Swazey. *The Courage to Fail: A Social View of Organ Transplants and Dialysis.* New Brunswick, NJ: Transaction, 2009.

Fox, Renee C., and Judith P. Swazey. *Spare Parts: Organ Replacement in American Society.* New Brunswick, NJ: Transaction, 2013.

Frazier, O. H., and James K. Kirklin. *Mechanical Circulatory Support, Vol. 1.* ISHLT Monograph Series. Philadelphia: Elsevier, 2001.

Fye, W. Bruce. *Caring for the Heart: Mayo Clinic and the Rise of Specialization.* New York: Oxford University Press, 2015.

Gillam, James T. *Life and Death in the Central Highlands: An American Sergeant in the Vietnam War, 1968–1970.* Denton: University of North Texas Press, 2010.

Greenberg, Daniel S. *Science, Money, and Politics: Political Triumph and Ethical Erosion.* Chicago: University of Chicago Press, 2001.

Heaman, E. A., Alison Li, and Shelley McKellar, eds. *Essays in Honour of Michael Bliss: Figuring the Social.* Toronto: University of Toronto Press, 2008.

Houghton, Peter. *On Death, Dying and Not Dying.* London: Jessica Kingsley, 2001.

Institute of Medicine. *The Artificial Heart: Prototypes, Policies, and Patients.* Washington, DC: National Academy Press, 1991.

Jeffrey, Kirk. *Machines in Our Hearts: The Cardiac Pacemaker, the Implantable Defibrillator, and American Health Care.* Baltimore: Johns Hopkins University Press, 2001.

Lasby, Clarence G. *Eisenhower's Heart Attack: How Ike Beat Heart Disease and Held On to the Presidency.* Lawrence: University Press of Kansas, 1997.

Lerner, Barron H. *When Illness Goes Public: Celebrity Patients and How We Look at Medicine.* Baltimore: Johns Hopkins University Press, 2006.

Liotta, Domingo. *The Amazing Adventures of a Heart Surgeon: The Artificial Heart: The Frontiers of Human Life.* Lincoln, NE: iUniverse, 2007.

Marcus Aurelius. *Meditations.* Translated by George Long. Sioux Falls, SD: NuVision, 2008.

Mattox, Kenneth L., ed. *The History of Surgery in Houston.* Austin, TX: Eakin Press, 1998.

McIngvale, Jim, with Thomas N. Duening and John M. Ivancevich. *How Mattress Mack's Uncompromising Attitude Built the Biggest Single Retail Store in America.* Chicago: Dearborn Trade, 2002.

McKellar, Shelley. *Artificial Hearts: The Allure and Ambivalence of a Controversial Medical Technology.* Baltimore: Johns Hopkins University Press, 2018.

McRae, Donald. *Every Second Counts: The Race to Transplant the First Human Heart.* London: Pocket Books, 2007.

Miller, G. Wayne. *King of Hearts: The True Story of the Maverick Who Pioneered Open Heart Surgery*. New York: Times Books, 2000.

Minetree, Harry. *Cooley: The Career of a Great Heart Surgeon*. New York: Harper's Magazine Press, 1973.

Monagan, David, with David O. Williams. *Journey into the Heart: A Tale of Pioneering Doctors and Their Race to Transform Cardiovascular Medicine*. New York: Gotham Books, 2007.

National Heart and Lung Institute, Artificial Heart Assessment Panel. *The Totally Implantable Artificial Heart: Economic, Ethical, Legal, Medical, Psychiatric [and] Social Implications: A Report*. Reprints from the collection of the University of Michigan Library. San Bernardino, CA: Prepared for Publishing by HP, 2017.

National Heart, Lung and Blood Institute. *The Artificial Heart: Planning for Evolving Technologies*. Washington, DC: NHLBI, 1994.

Ness, Roberta B. *Genius Unmasked*. New York: Oxford University Press, 2013.

The President's Commission on Heart Disease, Cancer and Stroke. *Report to the President: A National Program to Conquer Heart Disease, Cancer, and Stroke (Reports of the Subcommittees on Heart Disease, Cancer, and Stroke)*. Washington, DC: U.S. Government Printing Office, 1965.

Rothman, David J. *Strangers at the Bedside: A History of How Law and Bioethics Transformed Medical Decision Making*. Lexington, MA: Basic Books, 1991.

Salvaggio, John E. *New Orleans' Charity Hospital: A Story of Physicians, Politics, and Poverty*. Baton Rouge: Louisiana State University Press, 1992.

Schwartz, William B. *Life Without Disease: The Pursuit of Medical Utopia*. Berkeley: University of California Press, 1998.

Sharp, Lesley A. *Strange Harvest: Organ Transplants, Denatured Bodies, and the Transformed Self*. Berkeley: University of California Press, 2006.

Shaw, Margery, ed. *After Barney Clark: Reflections on the Utah Artificial Heart Program*. Austin: University of Texas Press, 1984.

Smolin, Shirley Karp. *Where the Heart Is*. Blurb Creative Publishing, 2012.

Spingarn, Natalie Davis. *Heartbeat: The Politics of Health Research*. Washington, DC: Robert B. Luce, 1976.

Strickland, Stephen P. *Politics, Science, and Dread Disease*. Cambridge, MA: Harvard University Press, 1972.

Texas Heart Institute Foundation. *Twenty-Five Years of Excellence: A History of the Texas Heart Institute*. Houston: Texas Heart Institute Foundation, 1989.

Thompson, Thomas. *Hearts*. London: Pan Books, 1972.

Westaby, Stephen. *Landmarks in Cardiac Surgery*. Oxford: Isis Medical Media, 1997.

Winters, William L., Jr., with Betsy Parrish. *Houston Hearts*. Houston, TX: Elisha Freeman, 2014.

INTERVIEW TRANSCRIPTS AND PAPERS

Michael E. DeBakey Papers: Profiles in Science, U.S. National Library of Medicine, https://profiles.nlm.nih.gov/ps/retrieve/Narrative/FJ/p-nid/322.

Oral History Interview of Dr. Michael E. DeBakey by David McComb, History of Medicine Division of the National Library of Medicine, June 29, 1969.

Mary Lasker Papers, "Mary Lasker and the Growth of the National Institutes of Health," Profiles in Science, U.S. National Library of Medicine, https://profiles.nlm.nih.gov/ps/retrieve/Narrative/TL/p-nid/200.

Dave Thompson and Chris Nelson, transcripts of interviews for O. H. "Bud" Frazier tribute film, August–October 2013.

JOURNAL ARTICLES

Abou-Awdi, Nancy L. "Thermo Cardiosystems Left Ventricular Assist Device as a Bridge to Cardiac Transplant." *AACN Journals* 2, no. 3 (August 1991).

Agustin, Gary C. "Ethical Issues Related to the Artificial Heart." *Journal of Religion and Health* 25, no. 3 (Fall 1986).

Annas, George J. "Consent to the Artificial Heart: The Lion and the Crocodiles." *Hastings Center Report* 13, no. 2 (April 1983).

Berenson, Claudia K., and Bernard I. Grosser. "Total Artificial Heart Implantation." *Archives of General Psychiatry* 41 (September 1984).

Butler, K. C., J. C. Moise, and R. K. Wampler. "The Hemopump—A New Cardiac Prosthesis Device." *IEEE Transactions on Biomedical Engineering*, 37, no. 2 (February 1990): 193–196.

Caplan, Arthur L. "The Artificial Heart." *Hastings Center Report* 12, no. 1 (1982): 22–24.

Cohn, William E., Daniel L. Timms, and O. H. Frazier. "Total Artificial Hearts: Past, Present, and Future." *Nature Reviews Cardiology* 12 (2015): 609–617.

Cooley, Denton, et al. "Total Artificial Heart in Two Staged Cardiac Transplantation." *Cardiovascular Disease* 3, no. 3 (September 1981): 305–319.

Cooley, Denton. "A Brief History of the Texas Heart Institute." *Texas Heart Institute Journal* 35, no. 3 (June 2008): 235–239.

DeBakey, Michael E. "The Artificial Heart: Total Replacement." *Transplantation Proceedings* 3, no. 4 (December 1971): 1445–1448.

DeBakey, Michael E. "John Gibbon and the Heart-Lung Machine: A Personal Encounter and His Import for Cardiovascular Surgery." *Annals of Thoracic Surgery* 76 (2003): S2188–S2194.

Dennis, Clarence. "Present and Future of the Artificial Heart." *Biomaterials, Medical Devices, and Artificial Organs* 3, no. 2 (1975): 155–160.

Dhruva, Sanket, and Rita Redberg. "Medical Device Regulation: Time to Improve Performance." *PLOS Medicine*, July 2012.

Frazier, O. H. "Mechanical Circulatory Assist Device Development at the Texas Heart Institute: A Personal Perspective." *Journal of Thoracic and Cardiovascular Surgery* 147, no. 6 (June 2014): 1738–1744.

Frazier, O. H., et al. "The Total Artificial Heart: Where We Stand." *Cardiology* 101, nos. 1–3 (2004): 117–121.

Gemmato, Courtney J., et al. "Thirty-Five Years of Mechanical Circulatory Support at the Texas Heart Institute." *Texas Heart Institute Journal* 32, no. 2 (2005): 168–177.

Gideon, Gil. "The Artificial Heart Juggernaut." *Hastings Center Report* 19, no. 2 (March 1989): 24–32.

Gilbert, Robert E. "Eisenhower's 1955 Heart Attack." *Politics and the Life Sciences* 27, no. 1 (2008): 2–21.

Jarvik, Robert K. "The Total Artificial Heart." *Scientific American*, January 1981, 74–80.

Jauhar, Sandeep. "The Artificial Heart." *New England Journal of Medicine* 350 (February 2004): 542–544.

Jonsen, Albert R. "The Artificial Heart's Threat to Others." *Hastings Center Report* 16, no. 1 (February 1986): 9–11.

Kolff, Willem. "Delays by Recalcitrant FDA, Reluctant NIH, and Fearful Industry: The Cost in Human Life, Happiness, Money, and Loss of Opportunity for American Industry." *Artificial Organs* 17, no. 9 (February 1993): 753–757.

Lubeck, Deborah P., and John P. Bunker. "Case Study #9: The Artificial Heart: Cost, Risks, and Benefits." *The Implications of Cost-Effectiveness Analysis of Medical Technology*, Office of Technology Assessment, May 1982.

Makower, J., A. Meer, and L. Denend. "FDA Impact on U.S. Medical Technology Innovation: A Survey of over 200 Medical Technology Companies." November 2010.

McKellar, Shelley. "Negotiating Risk: The Failed Development of Atomic Hearts in America, 1967–1977." *Technology and Culture* 54, no. 1 (January 2013): 1–39.

Messerli, Franz H., Adrian W. Messerli, and Thomas F. Lüscher. "Eisenhower's Billion-Dollar Heart Attack—50 Years Later." *New England Journal of Medicine* 353 (September 22, 2005): 1205–1207.

Miller, Leslie W., et al. "Use of a Continuous-Flow Device in Patients Awaiting Heart Transplantation." *New England Journal of Medicine* 357 (August 30, 2007): 885–896.

Roberts, William C. "Michael Ellis DeBakey: A Conversation with the Editor." *American Journal of Cardiology* 79, no. 7 (April 1, 1997): 929–950.

Roberts, William C. "Denton Arthur Cooley, MD: A Conversation with the Editor." *American Journal of Cardiology*, 79, no. 8 (April 15, 1997): 1078–1091.

Rose, Eric, et al. "Long-Term Use of a Left Ventricular Assist Device for End-Stage

Heart Failure." *New England Journal of Medicine* 345 (November 15, 2001): 1435–1443.

Stein, Amanda D. "The Heart's Surgeon." *TMC Pulse* 36, no. 7 (May 7, 2014): 13–15.

Strauss, Michael J. "The Political History of the Artificial Heart." *New England Journal of Medicine* 310 (February 2, 1984): 332–336.

MAGAZINE ARTICLES

"Artificial Heart Surgeon William Devries Transplants Himself to Greener Pastures." *People*, August 20, 1984.

Bailey, Ronald, and Alex Kerr. "A Patient's Gift to the Future of Heart Repair." *Life*, May 6, 1966, 84–92.

Baum, Dan. "No Pulse: How Doctors Reinvented the Human Heart." *Popular Science*, March 2012, 37–45, 74.

Baumgold, Julie. "In the Kingdom of the Brain." *New York Magazine*, February 6, 1989, 36–43.

Bernstein, Barton J. "The Artificial Heart Program." *Center Magazine*, May/June 1981, 22–41.

Clark, Matt. "A Tiny Booster for the Heart," *Newsweek*, May 16, 1988, 73.

Gonzales, Laurence. "The Rock 'n' Roll Heart of Robert Jarvik, Creator of the Artificial Heart." *Playboy*, April 1986.

Groopman, Jerome. "Heart Surgery, Unplugged." *New Yorker*, January 11, 1999, 43–51.

Groopman, Jerome. "Print Thyself." *New Yorker*, November 24, 2014.

Levy, Renee Gearthart. "The Beat Goes On." *Syracuse University Magazine* 5, no. 4 (1989).

McMurran, Kristin. "There's Nothing Artificial About the Way Robert Jarvik's Heart Beats for His Brainy Bride to Be." *People*, July 27, 1987.

Neill, Michael J., and Karen Roebuck. "Cardiac Arrest." *People*, September 14, 1992, 75–76.

Salter, James. "Two Great Surgical Teams Race for the Man-Made Heart." *Life*, September 1981, 34–36.

Sapolsky, Harvey M. "Here Comes the Artificial Heart." *The Sciences*, December 1978, 25–27.

Siebert, Charles. "The Rehumanization of the Heart: What Doctors Have Forgotten, Poets Have Always Known." *Harper's Magazine*, February 1990, 53–59.

Smith, William Michael. "Rock 'n' Roll Heart." *Oberlin Alumni Magazine*, Winter 2012.

Stipp, David. "New Hope for the Heart." *Fortune*, June 24, 1996.

Swartz, Mimi. "It Can't All Be Energy." *Texas Monthly*, November 11, 2017.

Thompson, Thomas. "The Texas Tornado vs. Dr. Wonderful." *Life*, April 10, 1970, 62B–74.

Thompson, Thomas. "The Year They Changed Hearts: A New and Disquieting Look at Transplants." *Life*, September 17, 1971, 56–70.

Wheelwright, Jeff. "Bill's Heart: The Troubling Story Behind a Historic Experiment." *Life*, May 1985, 33–43.

Yeaple, Judith Anne. "The Bionic Heart." *Popular Science*, April 1992, 65–69.

NEWSPAPER ARTICLES

Ackerman, Todd. "Baylor Honors Pioneer DeBakey with Library, Museum." *Houston Chronicle*, May 14, 2010.

Ackerman, Todd. "Legendary Heart Surgeons DeBakey, Cooley Mend Rift." *Houston Chronicle,* November 6, 2007.

Ackerman, Todd. "St. Luke's Exploring Hospital Sale Options." *Houston Chronicle*, November 3, 2012.

Ackerman, Todd. "St. Luke's to Sell to National Catholic System." *Houston Chronicle*, April 19, 2013.

Altman, Lawrence K. "Artificial Heart in Turmoil." *New York Times*, May 17, 1988.

Altman, Lawrence K. "The Feud." *New York Times*, November 27, 2007.

Altman, Lawrence K. "The Man on the Table Devised the Surgery." *New York Times*, December 25, 2006.

Altman, Lawrence K. "Third Patient Will Get Artificial Heart Sunday." *New York Times*, February 16, 1985.

Altman, Lawrence K. "A Tiny Heart Pump Saves Its First Life, Researchers Report." *New York Times*, May 5, 1988.

Associated Press. "Artificial Heart Survivor Stricken with Pneumonia." *Evening Star*, April 8, 1969.

Associated Press. "Heart Man Dies on 4th Day." *Daily News*, April 8, 1969.

Associated Press. "His Wife Pleads for a Heart to Replace Artificial Pump." *Daily News*, April 6, 1969.

Associated Press. "Patient with Artificial Heart Called Alert, Donor Sought." *Washington Star,* April 6, 1969.

Associated Press. "Plastic Heart Recipient Alert: Wife Issues Plea for Donor." *Hartford Courant*, April 6, 1969, 4A.

Associated Press. "Texas Plea Made for Heart Donor," *New York Times*, April 6, 1969.

Associated Press. "Total Artificial Heart Is Implanted in Man." *Evening Star*, April 4, 1969.

Balz, Dan. "Houston Surgeon in Trouble for Implanting Plastic Heart." *Washington Post*, August 9, 1981.

Berger, Eric. "Donor Brings Inventor of Artificial Heart Closer to Houston." *Houston Chronicle*, January 14, 2013.

Bernstein, Barton J. "Organs, Medicine, Business: The Artificial Heart in a Broader Context." *Sun-Sentinel*, December 7, 1986.

Bloom, Mark. "Heart Feud Grows: Cooley Aide Got U.S. Funds." *Daily News*, April 9, 1969.

Bowsher, Melodie. "Top Surgeons' Feud over Artificial Heart Boils on in Houston." *Wall Street Journal*, June 29, 1969.

Brauer, Ralph. "The Promise That Failed." *New York Times*, August 28, 1988.

Broad, William J. "Dr. Clark's Heart: A Story of Modern Marketing as Well as Modern Medicine." *New York Times*, March 20, 1983.

Chen, Edwin. "Artificial Heart—A Case of Pushing Science 'Too Fast.'" *Los Angeles Times*, January 12, 1990.

Clayton, James E. "Heart Transplants—The Legal and Ethical Issues." *Washington Post*, August 16, 1969, A10.

Dalton, Trent. "BiVACOR Artificial Heart: Daniel Timms Stroke of Genius." *The Australian*, March 7, 2015.

DeBakey, Michael. "Former Lake Charles Student Writes Story About Old Strasbourg." *American Press*, February 21, 1936.

"The Dracula of Medical Technology." *New York Times*, May 16, 1988.

Edson, Lee. "The Search for a 'Bionic' Heart." *New York Times*, October 21, 1979, SM10.

Feldman, Claudia. "Mike Templeton's Broken Heart." *Houston Chronicle*, April 12, 1992, 6–9, 14.

Felton, Keith S. "Heart Surgery, Its Heroes and Villains." *Los Angeles Times*, June 24, 1973.

"1st Mechanical Heart Man's Widow Sues." *Chicago Tribune*, April 17, 1971, 14.

Haberman, Clyde. "Artificial Hearts Ticking Along Decades After Jarvik-7 Debate." *New York Times*, March 20, 2016.

Hoffman, Ken. "'Mattress Mack' Slows Down, but He Still Works Harder than Most." *Houston Chronicle*, September 1, 2014.

"Houston Winning Mantle as Transplant Capital." *Washington Post*, August 4, 1968.

Hull, Tupper. "Man Dies Despite 3rd Heart." *Houston Chronicle*, August 3, 1981, 1A, 21A.

James, Ann. "Judge Dismisses Karp Jury, Rules for Drs. Cooley, Liotta." *Houston Chronicle*, June 30, 1972.

Kass, Miriam. "Man Given Mechanical Heart in First Total Replacement." *Houston Post*, April 5, 1969.

Kellum, B. F. "Artificial Heart: How Cooley Won Malpractice Suit." *Washington Post*, June 23, 1969, B4.

Loddeke, Leslie. "Heart Patient Pumped About Release." *Houston Chronicle*, September 1, 1992, A1, A8.

News Syndicate Co. "Use of Artificial Heart by Surgeon Is Probed." *Daily News*, April 9, 1969.

Nolte, Robert. "Heart Plant's Widow Tells Her Feelings." *Chicago Tribune*, April 10, 1969, B5.

Palomo, Juan Ramon. "Heart Patient from Holland Having Setback." *Houston Post*, August 2, 1981.

Raji, Bayan. "Texas Heart Institute Says St. Luke's Agreement 'Not Feasible." *Houston Business Journal*, May 17, 2013.

Randall, Judith. "Transplants, Apollo Both Misguided?" *Washington Star,* January 2, 1969.

Rich, Jan. "Cooley Implants Artificial Heart Here After Bypass Fails." *Houston Chronicle*, July 24, 1981.

Rich, Jan. "Designer of Artificial Organ Is Resigning from Heart Institute." *Houston Chronicle*, July 29, 1981.

Robertson, Kathy. "Kriton Medical Sues Doctor, Alleges Breach of Contract." *Sacramento Business Journal*, February 16, 2001.

Rosenfeld, Albert. "The Second Genesis: The Coming Control of Life." *Washington Post*, June 23, 1969, B4.

Russell, Cristine. "Clark's Case Impels FDA to Review Heart Program." *Washington Post*, December 18, 1982, A2.

Schier, Mary Jane. "Cooley Implants Artificial Heart." *Houston Chronicle,* July 24, 1981, 1A, 17A.

Schier, Mary Jane. "Dutchman Clings to Life as Doctors Seek Heart Donor." *Houston Post*, July 25, 1981, 1A, 28A.

Schier, Mary Jane. "Man with Plastic Heart Gets Real One." *Houston Post*, July 26, 1981.

Schmeck, Harold M. "Dr. Cooley Defends His Use of Artificial Heart." *New York Times*, April 10, 1969.

Scott, Janny. "Lack of Recognition Embitters Some Pioneers of Artificial Heart Design." *Los Angeles Times*, January 4, 1987.

"Senators Doctors Kennedy and Hatch." *New York Times*, July 15, 1988.

Smith, William Michael. "Doctor Doctor." *Houston Press*, August 25–31, 2011, 43.

SoRelle, Ruth. "Tiny Pump Used on First Heart Patient." *Houston Chronicle*, May 4, 1988, 8, 20.

Tribune Wire Services. "Karp Doctor Denies Violating U.S. Rules." *Chicago Tribune*, April 10, 1969, B5.

United Press International. "Heart Device Like Rival's, Cooley Admits." *Los Angeles Times*, June 29, 1972.

United Press International. "Widow Praises Artificial Heart Try That Failed." *Hartford Courant*, September 21, 1969, 4B.

Van Leer, Twila. "Doctors Look Back on Drama of Clark Heart Experiment." *Deseret News*, November 29, 1992.

Wampler, Richard K. "Tiny Experimental Pump Offers Hope for Heart Patients." *Los Angeles Times*, August 1, 1988.

Wilson, D. J. "Portable Heart Assist Pump Working Fine." *Houston Chronicle*, October 2, 1991, A1, A12.

VIDEOS

"Bud Frazier and Billy Cohn at TEDMED 2012," posted May 10, 2012, YouTube, https://www.youtube.com/watch?v=64-QTOUGNSk.

Grubin, David. *The Mysterious Human Heart: The Body's Perpetual Motion Machine.* Thirteen/WNET. Ambrose Video Publishing, 2007.

Nova. "Electric Heart." December 21, 1999. Transcript: http://www.pbs.org/wgbh/nova/transcripts/2617eheart.html.

Project Bionics Pioneer Interviews. Richard Wampler, Jean Kantrowitz, O. H. Frazier, Victor L. Poirier. https://asaio.com/about-us/asaio-pioneer-interviews.

WEB ARTICLES

Brennan, Imogen. "The Artificial Heart That Could Replace Transplants." Australia Unlimited, February 16, 2017. https://www.australiaunlimited.com/technology/danieltimms.

CBS News. "The Evolution of Artificial Hearts." January 31, 2002. https://www.cbsnews.com/news/the-evolution-of-artificial-hearts.

Genes, Nicholas. "Paul Winchell and the Artificial Heart." Medgadget, July 2005. https://www.medgadget.com/2005/07/paul_winchell_a.html.

MassDevice Staff. "Medical Device Makers Spend Millions to Meet FDA Rules, Study Finds." MedCityNews, November 19, 2010. https://medcitynews.com/2010/11/medical-device-makers-spend-millions-to-meet-fda-rules-study-finds.

National Library of Medicine, National Institutes of Health. "A Chronology of the National Heart, Lung, and Blood Institute Artificial Heart Program and Related Events." 1991. https://www.ncbi.nlm.nih.gov/books/NBK234439.

O'Brien, Alex. "How to Mend a Broken Heart." Mosaic, June 1, 2015. https://mosaicscience.com/story/artificial-heart.

Palomino, Joaquin. "The Heart Is Just a Pump." Verge, November 4, 2015. https://www.theverge.com/2015/11/4/9665902/artificial-heart-transplant-cedars-sinai-clinical-trials.

Ristich, Katharine. "The Last 5 Months of a Fighter: Remembering Robert Tools." Medscape, December 3, 2001. https://www.medscape.com/viewarticle/783837.

INDEX

INDEX

Heart disease, 21–23, 26–27, 29, 41,
43, 49, 75, 77, 78, 90, 92, 98–100,
108, 142, 148, 156, 158, 195, 238,
248
Heart failure, 22
Heart-lung machine, 34, 42, 43, 71–
74, 81, 82, 96, 104, 118, 124, 157,
181, 186–188, 206, 227
Heart monitor, 42
Heart transplants, 15, 22, 23, 43,
75–77, 79, 81–89, 92, 103–106,
109–111, 125–126, 131–133, 143–
145, 147, 148, 277
Heartbeat, 25
HeartMate I, 112, 145, 147
HeartMate II, 176, 195–198, 200, 206,
212, 224, 257, 277
Hearts (Thompson), 58
Hemolysis, 149, 171
Hemopump, 161–163, 173–174, 176,
182, 216, 244, 246, 260, 261
Henry, Butch, 18
Hippocratic oath, 120
Hofheinz, Roy, 183
Houston Chronicle, 143, 145
Humana, 139, 169
Hypothermia, 42
Hypoxia, 124

IBM Corporation, 72
Idiopathic cardiomyopathy, 142–143
Immune system, 105, 106
Impellers, 245, 257
Incident of the Yucatan Mini Pigs,
The, 17
Institutional Review Boards, 137, 138
International Society for Heart and
Lung Transplantation, 220

International Surgical Society, 85
Intrauterine devices (IUDs), 110, 124,
182
Itinerant surgery, 48–49

Jarvik-7 heart, 129–135, 138, 148, 165,
169, 216, 246, 266
Jarvik-2000 heart, 168, 175–176, 200
Jarvik, Murray, 127
Jarvik, Robert, 18, 117, 126–130, 136,
137, 155, 156, 165–176, 182, 198,
200, 211, 215, 216, 217, 238, 240,
246, 267, 272, 276
Jefferson Davis Hospital, 67–68, 70
Jhin, Michael, 190–192
Johns Hopkins Hospital, 64–66,
68–70, 187
Johnson & Johnson, 163, 255, 258,
264
Johnson & Johnson Center for Device
Innovation, 274–275
Johnson, Lyndon Baines, 28, 61, 108
*Journal of the American Medical
Association*, 84
Junction, Texas, 31

Kantrowitz, Adrian, 76, 77, 84, 87, 99,
116
Kantrowitz, Jean, 116
Karp, Haskell, 94–96, 98, 99, 118,
120, 124, 125, 128, 267
Karp, Shirley, 94, 95, 118–119
Karr, Mary, 14, 253
Kennedy, Edward M., 154
Kennedy, Jacqueline, 89
Kennedy, John F., 38–39, 90, 153

ABOUT THE AUTHOR

MIMI SWARTZ is a longtime executive editor at *Texas Monthly*, and a two-time National Magazine Award winner and a four-time finalist. She is the coauthor of the national bestseller *Power Failure,* with Sherron Watkins, about the failures at Enron and her work has appeared in *Vanity Fair, The New Yorker, Esquire,* and *Slate,* and her op-ed pieces appear regularly in the *New York Times.*